O D L

OXFORD DIABETES LIBRARY

Diabetic Neuropathy

Edited by

Solomon Tesfaye

Honorary Professor of Diabetic Medicine,
University of Sheffield, and Consultant Physician,
Sheffield Teaching Hospitals,
Royal Hallamshire Hospital,
Sheffield, UK

Andrew Boulton

Professor of Medicine,
University of Manchester, and Consultant Physician,
Manchester Royal Infirmary,
Manchester, UK

OXFORD
UNIVERSITY PRESS

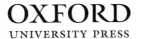

OXFORD
UNIVERSITY PRESS

Great Clarendon Street, Oxford OX2 6DP

Oxford University Press is a department of the University of Oxford.
It furthers the University's objective of excellence in research, scholarship,
and education by publishing worldwide in

Oxford New York

Auckland Cape Town Dar es Salaam Hong Kong Karachi
Kuala Lumpur Madrid Melbourne Mexico City Nairobi
New Delhi Shanghai Taipei Toronto

With offices in

Argentina Austria Brazil Chile Czech Republic France Greece
Guatemala Hungary Italy Japan Poland Portugal Singapore
South Korea Switzerland Thailand Turkey Ukraine Vietnam

Oxford is a registered trade mark of Oxford University Press
in the UK and in certain other countries

Published in the United States
by Oxford University Press Inc., New York

British Library Cataloguing in Publication Data

Data available

Library of Congress Cataloging in Publication Data

Data available

Typeset by Newgen Imaging Systems (P) Ltd., Chennai, India
Printed in Great Britain
on acid-free paper by
Ashford Colour Press Ltd., Gosport, Hampshire

ISBN 978–0–19–955106–4

10 9 8 7 6 5 4 3 2 1

Contents

Preface

Currently available books on Diabetic Neuropathy tend to be large reference texts and there is no pocket book with concise, summarized points for the clinician dealing with diabetic neuropathic patients. Diabetic neuropathy is very common affecting up to 50 % of all diabetic patients and can result in disabling neuropathic pain, lower extremity amputations and troublesome autonomic neuropathies (gastroparesis, erectile dysfunction, sudden cardiac death etc.). With the rising prevalence of diabetes the prevalence of neuropathy is likely to increase. Having lectured to GPs and specialists nationally and internationally we have come to realise that there is a need for an small, up-to-date book that summarizes key points in the diagnosis and appropriate management of the various clinical presentations of diabetic neuropathy.

The book aims to be primarily a reference aid to the busy, practicing clinician managing neuropathic patients. Many doctors will have little time to read about the varied conditions they have to deal with and hence this book has been made deliberately concise with plenty of bullet points, illustrations and protocols for management. Each Chapter has been written by authorities in the area and the topics have been carefully selected to address essential areas in diabetic neuropathy.

We do hope this book will be useful to clinicians that deal with the varied presentations of diabetic neuropathy including: diabetologists, general physicians, neurologists, junior doctors, general practitioners, diabetes specialist nurses, practice nurses, clinical research fellows, podiatrists, clinical scientists, and pain specialists.

Solomon Tesfaye
Andrew JM Boulton

Contributors

Andrew J M Boulton
University of Manchester,
Manchester Royal Infirmary,
Manchester, UK

Frank L Bowling
Manchester Royal Infirmary,
University Department
of Medicine, Manchester, UK

Hassan Fadavi
Cardiovascular Research
Group, Division of
Cardiovascular and Endocrine
Sciences, University of
Manchester, Manchester, UK

Roy Freeman
Center for Autonomic and
Peripheral Nerve Disorders,
Beth Israel Deaconess
Medical Center, Boston,
Massachusetts, USA

Rayaz A Malik
Cardiovascular Research
Group, Division of
Cardiovascular and Endocrine
Sciences, University of
Manchester, Manchester, UK

David E Price
Diabetes Centre, Morriston
Hospital, Swansea, Wales, UK

Jonathan Shaw
Baker IDI
Heart and Diabetes Institute,
Melbourne, Australia

Robyn Tapp
International Public Health Unit,
Monash University, Australia

Mitra Tavakoli
Cardiovascular Research Group,
Division of Cardiovascular and
Endocrine Sciences,
University of Manchester,
Manchester, UK

Solomon Tesfaye
University of Sheffield,
Sheffield Teaching Hospitals,
Royal Hallamshire Hospital,
Sheffield, UK

Symbols and abbreviations

↓	decreased
↑	increased
ACE	angiotensin converting enzyme
ADA	American Diabetes Association
AGEs	advanced glycation end products
ARs	aldose reductase
ARIs	AR inhibitors
as	axonal sprouts
rhBDNF	brain-derived neurotrophic factor
CASE	computer-aided sensory examination
CCM	confocal corneal microscopy
CRP	C-reactive protein
CSF	Cerebro-spinal fluid
CT	computed tomography
DAG	1,2-diacylglycerol
DCCT	Diabetes Control and Complications Trial
DL-DOPS	DL and L-dihydroxyphenylserine
DPAN	diabetic peripheral autonomic neuropathy
DPN	diabetic peripheral neuropathy
ECG	electrocardiogram
EP	electrophysiology
ESR	erythrocyte sedimentation rate
fMRI	functional MRI
FREMS	frequency-modulated electromagnetic neural stimulation
HIV	human immunodeficiency virus
IENF	intra-epidermal nerve fibre
KDM	known diabetes mellitus
MMP	matrix metalloproteinase
MRI	magnetic resonance imaging
MRS	magnetic resonance spectroscopy
MRSA	methicillin resistant *Staphylococcus aureus*

NCS	nerve conduction studies
NCV	nerve conduction velocity
NGF	nerve growth factor
NNH	number needed to harm
NNT	number needed to treat
NSS	neuropathy symptom score
OGTT	oral glucose tolerance test
PDN	painful diabetic neuropathy
PKC	protein kinase C
QST	quantitative sensory testing
RCT	random clinical trial
RCW	removable cast walkers
SDH	sorbitol dehydrogenase
SNRI	serotonin noradrenaline re-uptake inhibitor
TCA	tricyclic antidepressants
TCC	total contact casts
TENS	transcutaneous electrical stimulation
UKPDS	United Kingdom Prospective Diabetes Study
uscp	unassociated Schwann cell profiles
VACSDM	VA cooperative study on Type 2 diabetes mellitus
VPT	vibration perception threshold

Chapter 1

Epidemiology of diabetic neuropathy

Robyn Tapp and Jonathan Shaw

> **Key points**
> - Diabetic neuropathies affect up to 50% of those with diabetes.
> - The most common form is peripheral diabetic neuropathy.
> - Peripheral diabetic neuropathy is present in around 30% of those treated in a clinic setting.
> - The key treatable risk factor for peripheral diabetic neuropathy is glycaemic control.
> - An understanding of diabetic neuropathies is vital for improved targeting and treatment of high risk groups.

1.1 Introduction

Diabetic neuropathies affect up to 50% of those with diabetes. They encompass a range of conditions affecting the nervous system, of which the most common forms are peripheral and autonomic neuropathies. This chapter will focus on the epidemiology and risk factors for peripheral neuropathy which is the leading long-term complication of diabetes, with some background detail on autonomic neuropathy. Diabetic peripheral neuropathy (DPN) is defined as 'the presence of symptoms and/or signs of peripheral nerve dysfunction in people with diabetes after the exclusion of other causes' (1). Assessment can only be made by undertaking a clinical examination as peripheral neuropathy is very often asymptomatic. DPN is a major contributor to foot ulcers and amputation. Given the high cost (both economic and personal) of treating foot ulcers, it is important that we understand the modifiable risk factors associated with the development of neuropathy, in order to delay or prevent its development.

1.2 **Definition of DPN**

International recommendations (1; 2) have been developed for the diagnosis of peripheral neuropathy (Box 1.1). These recommendations require that at least one measure from each of the following categories should be included: clinical symptoms, clinical signs, neurophysiology, quantitative sensory testing, and autonomic function tests. Simple assessment of neuropathy is possible. For example, large nerve fibre function can be assessed in the foot with a 128-Hz tuning fork, monofilaments and by examining ankle reflexes, while pinprick sensation and hot and cold rods can be used to assess small nerve fibre function Autonomic neuropathy can be assessed using postural changes in blood pressure, and symptoms of neuropathy can be assessed using a simple validated questionnaire such as the neuropathy symptom score (NSS). The NSS includes questions about numbness and tingling in the feet and toes. Neuropathy using these assessment tools would be defined as present if two or more of the four areas of assessment were abnormal (3).

1.3 **Prevalence of DPN**

Accurate data on the prevalence of neuropathy have been difficult to acquire as there has been wide variability in the clinical tools used to define neuropathy and very few studies have been undertaken in population-based settings where estimates are less biased towards those with more severe disease. Additionally, only a limited number of studies have assessed neuropathy in populations defined by an oral glucose tolerance test (OGTT)—defining the total diabetic population. Few studies have included a sample from the general population with normal glucose tolerance, allowing for an accurate assessment of the degree that diabetes contributes to the development of peripheral neuropathy.

There is a great need for population-based studies, using standardized protocols, for meaningful estimates of the prevalence of DPN to be made. Nevertheless, some accurate estimates have now been established and the impact of the main confounding factors on prevalence has been assessed.

Box 1.1 Diagnostic tools to define peripheral neuropathy
A diagnosis of DPN should include assessment of
• Clinical symptoms
• Clinical signs
• Neurophysiology
• Quantitative sensory testing
• Autonomic neuropathy

1.4 Type 2 diabetes

Type 2 diabetes is the most common form of diabetes, making up ~90% of cases. The prevalence of peripheral neuropathy among those with known Type 2 diabetes in the clinic-based setting is ~30% and in population-based settings is ~20% (known diabetes mellitus (KDM)), with the prevalence ranging from 7.6% to 68.0% in clinic-based studies and 13.1% to 45.0% in population-based studies (Table 1.1) (4).

In studying the prevalence of complications among those with Type 2 diabetes, the setting is of great importance. Population-based studies, in which diabetes is defined by an OGTT, have provided more consistent prevalence estimates of peripheral neuropathy, though the prevalences have still varied by ~8% points. This setting is important as screening by OGTT identifies the total diabetic population. The prevalence observed in clinic-based populations is dependent on referral patterns and is biased towards those with more advanced disease. As an example, in a study by Cabezas-Cerrato *et al.*, the prevalence of peripheral neuropathy was determined in both the primary care and hospital clinic setting. The prevalence of peripheral neuropathy was 21% in the primary care setting and 27% in the hospital clinic patients (5).

In a national population-based study of Australia, the prevalence of neuropathy, defined as present if two or more of four scales were abnormal (the NSS, the neuropathy disability score, pressure perception test, and postural hypertension), was 13.1% among those with known diabetes and 7.1% among those with newly diagnosed diabetes (3). In two further population-based studies from Mauritius (6) and Egypt (7), the prevalences of neuropathy were 12.7% and 3.6% in Mauritius, and 21.9% and 13.6% in Egypt, among those with known and newly diagnosed diabetes, respectively. In contrast to these studies, the population-based 1999–2000 National Health and Nutrition Survey in the United States used self-report diabetes and defined peripheral neuropathy by self-report symptoms and monofilament sensitivity (8). In this study the prevalence of neuropathy was 28.5%—considerably higher than that identified in studies in which diabetes was defined by an OGTT and the diagnosis of neuropathy based on clinical assessment. In addition to the impact of not defining

Table 1.1 Prevalence of DPN among those with Type 2 diabetes

	Median prevalence	Inter-quartile range	Range
Peripheral neuropathy			
Clinic-based studies	28.8	20.0–38.3	7.6–68.0
Population-based studies	24.1	17.2–32.4	13.1–45.0

diabetes by an OGTT, the inconsistent use of diagnostic tools to classify complications has been shown to dramatically affect the prevalence reported and this may account for the higher prevalence observed in this study. To provide some insight into the impact of definition on the prevalence of neuropathy, the Diabetes Control and Complications Trial (DCCT) compared the prevalence of neuropathy using 11 different definitions and showed that in one population the prevalence varied from 0.3% using a sensory examination through to 21.8% using nerve conduction tests.

1.5 Type 1 diabetes

The prevalence of peripheral neuropathy among those with Type 1 diabetes in the clinic-based setting overall is around 26%, with the prevalence ranging from 3.0% to 65.8% in clinic-based settings and from 12.8% to 54.0% in population-based studies (Table 1.2) (4).

The prevalence of DPN among those with Type 1 diabetes has been best described in the EURODIAB complications study, which examined 3250 randomly selected patients with Type 1 diabetes from 31 centres in 16 European countries (9). Neuropathy was defined as present when two or more of the following criteria were met: [1] the presence of one or more symptoms, [2] absence of two or more ankle or knee reflexes, [3] abnormal vibration perception threshold, and [4] abnormal autonomic function (a postural fall in systolic BP of at least 30 mmHg and/or loss of heart rate variability (R-R ratio <1)). The overall prevalence of peripheral diabetic neuropathy was 28%. With the exception of five centres in which the prevalence was over 35%, there were no significant differences in the prevalence of neuropathy across centres/countries. The study authors suggested that the high prevalence in a few centres was more likely to have been a consequence of variation in the technique of neurological and neurophysiological examination, or possibly a consequence of differing referral patterns among those centres, rather than a true difference in prevalence.

Table 1.2 Prevalence of DPN among those with Type 1 diabetes			
	Median prevalence	**Inter-quartile range**	**Range**
Peripheral neuropathy			
Clinic-based studies	25.5	22.7–29.0	3.0–65.8
Population-based studies	†	†	12.8–54.0
† number of studies too limited to report accurate estimates.			

1.6 Risk factors for DPN

A number of studies both among those with Type 1 and Type 2 diabetes have assessed risk factors for peripheral neuropathy. The common underlying factors identified are glycaemic control, age, height, and duration of diabetes (3; 6; 7; 9), while other factors such as hypertension, ethnicity, smoking, microalbuminuria, dyslipidaemia, and hypoinsulinaemia have shown mixed results (3; 6; 7; 9–13).

The identification of untreated risk factors provides a basis for improved management of those with diabetes through the initiation and more aggressive treatment of modifiable factors. Studies both of cross-sectional and prospective design have identified the main modifiable risk factor for peripheral neuropathy as glycaemic control (3; 7; 9). The EURODIAB study showed that for each standard deviation increase in HbA1c, there was a 60% increased risk chance of having peripheral neuropathy (9). The DCCT, a randomized clinical trial designed to determine the impact of tight glycaemic control on the development of diabetes-related complications in Type 1 diabetes, showed that tight glycaemic control reduced the risk of developing clinical neuropathy by 60%–69% over 6.5 years. After the trial and the intensive intervention ended, the differences in HbA1c between the two arms of the study rapidly disappeared. However, the benefits (in relation to neuropathy and other complications) of being in the original tight glycaemic control group were still evident 8 years later (14), leading some to hypothesize that 'metabolic memory' may be an important factor in the development of diabetic neuropathy and other diabetic complications. Recent findings from a lifestyle intervention study designed to determine the impact of a lifestyle modification (diet and exercise) on painful neuropathy among those with impaired glucose tolerance suggest that tight glycaemic control may improve neuropathic symptoms (15). Further research is needed to confirm these findings.

The association between glycaemic control and peripheral neuropathy is less evident among those with Type 2 diabetes. The United Kingdom Prospective Diabetes Study (UKPDS) which was designed to examine the impact of intensive glycaemic control on the development of diabetes-related complications in Type 2 diabetes showed no consistent impact of glycaemic control on the development of neuropathy (16). It may be that neuropathy is not as closely related to glycaemic control as are other complications among people with Type 2 diabetes, or more plausibly the difference in definition of neuropathy may account for the differing findings. The UKPDS defined neuropathy as present by loss of both ankle or knee reflexes or mean biothesiometer reading from both big toes 25 V or greater, while the DCCT used a comprehensive definition of neuropathy.

...difiable risk factors in the observational setting have not ... associations with neuropathy among those with either ...ype 2 diabetes, nevertheless it is strongly recommended ...sion and lipids be well controlled and smoking ceased (1).

While risk factors such as height, sex, duration of diabetes, ethnicity, and age are not modifiable, they can be used to identify a group at high risk of DPN for early intervention. Several studies have identified a strong association with height (3; 6; 17). Height is associated with the length of axons and longer axons are more prone to metabolic disturbances (18). It is largely thought that the strong association between height and peripheral diabetic neuropathy may account for the higher prevalence of neuropathy observed in men compared to women. Duration of diabetes is a strong risk factor for neuropathy— using data from the AusDiab study as an example, for each 10 years of diabetes duration the risk of developing neuropathy increased 73% (3). With regard to ethnicity, it has been shown in a study by Abbott et al. that those of South Asian and African Caribbean ethnicity have a much lower prevalence of neuropathy and the subsequent foot ulcers and amputations compared to white Europeans (19). This study was unique in that the population were from the UK where healthcare is free and disparity due to access to health care were minimized. In contrast to this a study by Pradeepa et al. identified a crude prevalence of 26.1% among urban South Asians with Type 2 diabetes (20). Although it is difficult to compare across studies due the differences in methodology, this would appear to suggest the prevalence may not, in fact, be lower among South Asians compared with Europeans. Nevertheless, further research is needed to clarify ethnic differences.

1.7 **Summary**

Most of the financial costs associated with diabetes are related to the prevention and treatment of complications. DPN is the most common long-term complication of diabetes. It has been shown to affect ~30% of those seen in a clinic setting. There are a number of factors that can be used to identify those at high risk of developing neuropathy, including poor glycaemic control, height, and duration of diabetes. Furthermore, targeting the modifiable risk factors could potentially delay or prevent the development of neuropathy if aggressively treated. The costs of foot ulcers and amputations are extremely high and given the rising prevalence of diabetes, the burden of foot complications is likely to remain high. Throughout the world the prevalence of diabetes is reaching epidemic levels, and with this the number of people developing related complications will continue to rise. An understanding of the epidemiology of diabetic neuropathies is vital for improved targeting of treatment of high risk groups (Box 1.2).

Box 1.2 Epidemiology of diabetic neuropathy

Important underlying risk factors
- Glycaemic control
- Age
- Height
- Duration of diabetes

Other possible risk factors
- Hypertension
- Smoking
- Microalbuminuria
- Dyslipidaemia
- Hypoinsulinaemia
- Ethnicity

References

1. Boulton AJ, Vinik AI, Arezzo JC et al. Diabetic neuropathies: a statement by the American Diabetes Association. *Diabetes Care* 2005; **28**: 956–62.

2. American Diabetes Association, American Academy of Neurology. Report and Recommendations of the San Antonio Conference on Diabetic Neuropathy. *Diabetes Care* 1988; **11**: 592–7.

3. Tapp R, Shaw J, deCourten M, Dunstan D, Welborn T, Zimmet P. Foot complications in type 2 diabetes: an Australian population based study. *Diabet Med* 2003; **20**: 105–13.

4. Tapp R, Sicree R, Zimmet P, Shaw J. *The Global Burden. Diabetes and Impaired Glucose Tolerance. Complications of Diabetes*, 3rd edition. Gan D, Ed. International Diabetes Federation, Brussels, 2006; pp. 111–49.

5. Cabezas-Cerrato J. The prevalence of clinical diabetic polyneuropathy in Spain: a study in primary care and hospital clinic groups. Neuropathy Spanish Study Group of the Spanish Diabetes Society (SDS). *Diabetologia* 1998; **41**: 1263–9.

6. Shaw JE, Hodge AM, deCourten M et al. Diabetic neuropathy in Mauritius: prevalence and risk factors. *Diabet Res Clin Pract* 1998; **42**: 131–9.

7. Herman WH, Aubert RE, Engelgau MM et al. Diabetes mellitus in Egypt: glycaemic control and microvascular and neuropathic complications. *Diabet Med* 1998; **15**: 1045–51.

8. Gregg EW, Sorlie P, Paulose-Ram R et al. Prevalence of lower-extremity disease in the U.S. adult population ≥40 years of age with and without diabetes. *Diabetes Care* 2004; **27**: 1591–7.

9. Tesfaye S, Stevens L, Stephenson J et al. Prevalence of diabetic peripheral neuropathy and its relation to glycaemic control and potential risk factors: the EURODIAB IDDM Complications Study. *Diabetologia* 1996; **39**: 1377–84.

10. Adler AI, Boyko EJ, Ahroni JH, Stensel V, Forsberg RC, Smith DG. Risk factors for diabetic peripheral sensory neuropathy: results of the Seattle Prospective Diabetic Foot Study. *Diabetes Care* 1997; **20**: 1162–7.

11. Sands ML, Shetterly SM, Franklin GM, Hamman RF. Incidence of distal symmetric (sensory) neuropathy in NIDDM. The San Luis Valley Diabetes Study. *Diabetes Care* 1997; **20**: 322–9.

12. Partanen J, Niskanen L, Lehtinen J, Mervaala E, Siitonen O, Uusitupa M. Natural history of peripheral neuropathy in patients with non-insulin-dependent diabetes mellitus. *N Engl J Med* 1995; **333**: 89–94.

13. Davis TM, Yeap BB, Davis WA, Bruce DG (2008). Lipid-lowering therapy and peripheral sensory neuropathy in type 2 diabetes: Fremantle Diabetes Study. *Diabetologia,* **51**: 562–6.

14. Martin CL, Albers J, Herman WH *et al.* Neuropathy among the diabetes control and complications trial cohort 8 years after trial completion. *Diabetes Care* 2006; **29**: 340–4.

15. Smith AG, Russell J, Feldman EL *et al.* Lifestyle intervention for pre-diabetic neuropathy. *Diabetes Care* 2006; **29**: 1294–9.

16. UK Prospective Diabetes Study (UKPDS) Group. Intensive blood-glucose control with sulphonylureas or insulin compared with conventional treatment and risk of complications in patients with type 2 diabetes (UKPDS 33). *Lancet* 1998; **352**: 837–53.

17. Cheng YJ, Gregg EW, Kahn HS, Williams DE, De Rekeneire N, Narayan KM. Peripheral insensate neuropathy—a tall problem for US adults? *Am J Epidemiol* 2006; **164**: 873–80.

18. Gadia MT, Natori N, Ramos LB, Ayyar DR, Skyler JS, Sosenko JM. Influence of height on quantitative sensory, nerve-conduction, and clinical indices of diabetic peripheral neuropathy. *Diabetes Care* 1987; **10**: 613–6.

19. Abbott CA, Garrow AP, Carrington AL, Morris J, Van Ross ER, Boulton AJ. Foot ulcer risk is lower in South-Asian and African-Carribbean compared with European diabetic patients in the U.K. *Diabetes Care* 2005; **28**: 1869–75.

20. Pradeepa R, Rema M, Vignesh J, Deepa M, Deepa R, Mohan V. Prevalence and risk factors for diabetic neuropathy in an urban south Indian population: the Chennai Urban Rural Epidemiology Study (CURES-55). *Diabet Med* 2008; **19**: 19.

Chapter 2

Pathogenesis of human diabetic neuropathy

Mitra Tavakoli, Moaz Mojaddidi, Hassan Fadavi, and Rayaz A Malik

> **Key points**
> - The pathogenesis of human diabetic neuropathy is complex.
> - Experimental studies provide a mechanistic basis for nerve damage and repair.
> - Translational work in patients is limited and we have no effective treatment.
> - The basis of painful diabetic neuropathy is poorly understood.
> - The treatment of pain shows limited efficacy with considerable side effects.

2.1 Abstract

The underlying pathology and aetiology of the diabetic neuropathies are varied and complex. Data in animal models and in cell culture provide a conceptual framework for the cause and treatment of human diabetic neuropathy. However, due to limited translational work, much debate and controversy exist over the cause(s) and hence treatment of human diabetic neuropathy. To date we have no effective treatment(s) for human diabetic neuropathy. Similarly many mechanisms have been proposed for painful diabetic neuropathy (PDN), yet very few have been verified in diabetic patients.

2.2 Introduction

Data from animal models and cell culture provide a conceptual framework for the cause and treatment of diabetic neuropathy (1) (Figure 2.1). However, these damaging pathways established in animal models have not been verified in the patient and multiple interventions have failed in clinical trials (2).

Figure 2.1 Pathogenesis of diabetic neuropathy

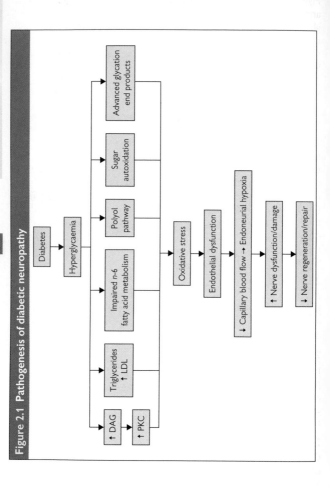

2.3 **Metabolic factors**

2.3.1 **Hyperglycaemia**

Hyperglycaemia is clearly important in the genesis of nerve damage and recent studies suggest that even minimal perturbations in blood glucose in those with impaired glucose tolerance (IGT) may lead to the development of small nerve fibre damage and neuropathic pain (3). Neuropathy improved in patients with Type 1 diabetes following intensive insulin treatment (Diabetes Control and Complications Trial (DCCT)) (4) and after pancreas transplantation (5). However, in the VA cooperative study on Type 2 diabetes mellitus (VACSDM) despite a 2.07% difference in HbA1c over 2 years there was no effect on neuropathy (6).

2.3.2 **Polyol pathway**

Increased flux through the polyol pathway via enhanced activity of its two key enzymes, aldose reductase (AR) and sorbitol dehydrogenase (SDH), leads to accumulation of sorbitol and fructose, respectively, and is associated with a reduction in nerve conduction velocity (NCV) (7). Blockade of this pathway with AR inhibitors (ARIs) ameliorates the NCV deficit consistently in experimental animals, yet a meta-analysis of 19 trials, testing four different ARIs between 4 and 208 weeks duration (median 24 weeks), demonstrated a small effect on motor NCV without benefit in sensory nerves (8).

2.3.3 **Myoinositol**

Myoinositol deficiency has also been proposed to play a role in the pathogenesis of diabetic neuropathy. However, nerve myoinositol levels do not differ in patients with normal glucose tolerance, IGT, and Type 2 diabetes (1).

2.3.4 **Glycation**

Hyperglycaemia results in the formation of advanced glycation end products (AGEs), which in turn act on specific receptors (RAGE) to activate, monocytes and endothelial cells, increasing the production of cytokines and adhesion molecules (9). However, there are no clinical trials showing efficacy to date in human diabetic neuropathy (2).

2.3.5 **Oxidative stress**

Oxidative stress is considered to be important in the pathogenesis of diabetic neuropathy in animal models. However, no long-term antioxidant treatment has established efficacy for human diabetic neuropathy (2).

2.4 **Vascular factors**

A large body of data implicates vascular disease in the pathogenesis of diabetic neuropathy.

2.4.1 **Angiotensin converting enzyme (ACE) inhibitors**

ACE inhibitors mediate increased endothelium-dependent vessel relaxation but also reduce AGE accumulation. In a double-blind placebo-controlled clinical trial, Trandolapril over 12 months improved motor NCV, M-wave amplitude, F-wave latency, and sural nerve amplitude (10).

2.4.2 **PKC-β inhibitors**

1,2-diacylglycerol (DAG) induced activation of protein kinase C (PKC); in particular, PKC-β has been proposed to play a major role in diabetic neuropathy (1). However, Phase III clinical trials have not demonstrated any benefit in diabetic patients with neuropathy (2).

2.4.3 **Hydroxymethylglutaryl CoA reductase inhibitor**

Although, hydroxymethylglutaryl CoA reductase inhibitors or statins work principally by reducing low-density lipoprotein levels, they also reduce AGE in diabetic patients and 2 years of simvastatin has shown a trend towards slower progression of neuropathy (11).

2.5 **Neurotrophins**

Neurotrophins promote the survival of specific neuronal populations by inducing morphological differentiation, enhancing nerve regeneration, stimulating neurotransmitter expression, and altering the physiological characteristics of neurones (12). Both nerve growth factor (NGF) (13) and brain-derived neurotrophic factor (rhBDNF) (14) have failed to demonstrate a significant benefit in patients with diabetic neuropathy.

2.5.1 **Painful Diabetic Neuropathy**

The pathophysiology of neuropathic pain in diabetic neuropathy is complex and not well understood. Central and peripheral mechanisms (Figure 2.2) have been proposed to generate neuropathic pain, yet many of the postulated abnormalities are derived principally from models of non-diabetic painful neuropathy and very few have been confirmed in diabetic patients.

Figure 2.2 Central and peripheral mechanisms of PDN

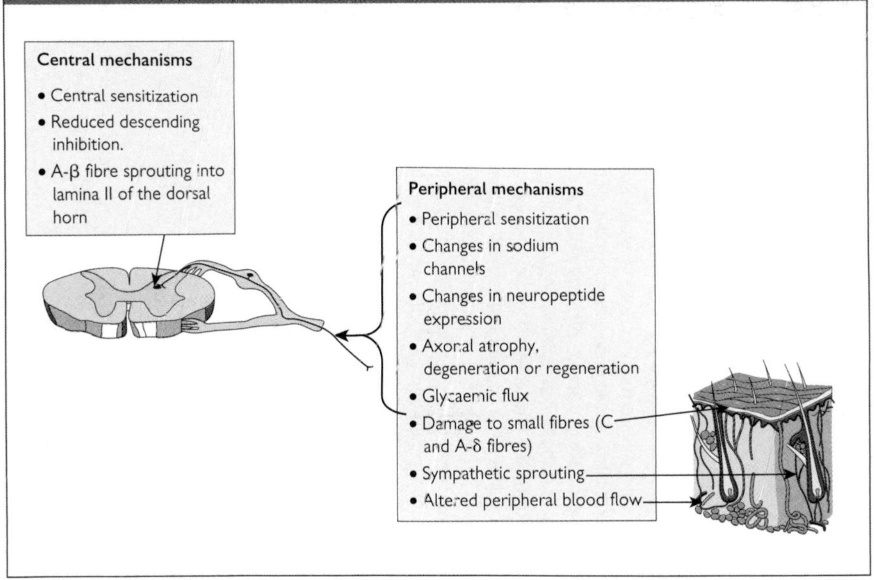

Central mechanisms
- Central sensitization
- Reduced descending inhibition.
- A-β fibre sprouting into lamina II of the dorsal horn

Peripheral mechanisms
- Peripheral sensitization
- Changes in sodium channels
- Changes in neuropeptide expression
- Axonal atrophy, degeneration or regeneration
- Glycaemic flux
- Damage to small fibres (C and A-δ fibres)
- Sympathetic sprouting
- Altered peripheral blood flow

2.6 **Peripheral mechanisms**

2.6.1 **Pathology**

It has been suggested that degenerating nerve fibres and those that exhibit impaired regeneration may generate inappropriate excitation impulses which are perceived as pain and paraesthesiae. Thus in sural nerve biopsies acute axonal degeneration and in particular small fibre regeneration have been suggested to lead to the development of PDN (Figure 2.3). In a skin biopsy study significant intra-epidermal nerve fibre (IENF, C-fibre) loss occurred in patients with PDN (15), yet in another study diabetic patients with and without PDN showed no difference in IENF density (16). This suggests that the basis of pain is likely to be complex.

2.6.2 **Hyperexcitability**

Hyperglycaemia leads to an increase in axonal excitability and a reduction in the refractory period in poorly controlled diabetic patients compared to well-controlled diabetic patients (HbA1c < 7%) and non-diabetic subjects. In diabetic neuropathy, ongoing damage results in hyperexcitability of primary afferent nociceptors (peripheral sensitization) characterized by a lowered activation threshold with an exaggerated response to a given stimulus, and abnormal spontaneous activity. Peripheral sensitization leads to hyperexcitability in central neurons (central sensitization) and generation of spontaneous impulses within the axon as well as the dorsal root ganglion of these peripheral nerves (17).

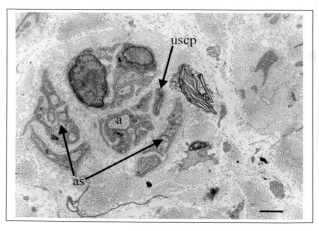

Figure 2.3 Electron micrograph of a sural nerve biopsy from a patient with diabetic neuropathy showing increased degeneration as evidenced by the presence of increased unassociated Schwann cell profiles (uscp) and regeneration in the form of axonal sprouts (as).

2.6.3 **Ion channels**

In chronic neuropathic pain, expression of a range of ion channels including sodium, potassium, and calcium channels is increased. Thus, along sites of nerve fibre injury sodium channels accumulate facilitating hyperexcitability, and discharge of ectopic electrical impulses contributes to the generation of electrical impulses to the dorsal horn (18).

2.6.4 **Sympathetic alterations**

Damaged peripheral nerves become epinephrine-sensitive and abnormal transmission of information from one axon to another via ephaptic transmission or 'cross-talk' leads to sympathetically mediated pain. Recent studies show impaired C-fibre-mediated vasoconstriction suggestive of inappropriate local blood flow regulation in the pathogenesis of pain in diabetic neuropathy (19).

2.6.5 **Central involvement**

Central changes at the level of the spinal cord are very important in the development and perception of neuropathic pain (20). When peripheral nerves are injured, local sympathetic fibres sprout terminals that surround large afferent A fibres which release substance P generating signals that may be misinterpreted as mechanical allodynia.

2.7 **Conclusions**

Whilst the pathogenesis of nerve damage and the development of pain are established in experimental states, the processes resulting in human diabetic neuropathy remain poorly studied and hence treatment at present is limited to symptomatic treatment.

References

1. Tomlinson DR, Gardiner NJ. Glucose neurotoxicity. *Nat Rev Neurosci* 2008; **9**: 36–45.

2. Ziegler D. Treatment of diabetic neuropathy and neuropathic pain: how far have we come? *Diabetes Care* 2008; **31**: S255–61.

3. Smith AG, Singleton JR. Impaired glucose tolerance and neuropathy. *Neurologist* 2008; **14**(1): 23–29.

4. DCCT Trial Research Group. The effect of intensive diabetes therapy on the development and progression of neuropathy. *Ann Int Med* 1995; **122**: 561–8.

5. Mehra S, Tavakoli M, Kallinikos PA *et al.* Corneal confocal microscopy detects early nerve regeneration after pancreas transplantation in patients with type 1 diabetes. *Diabetes Care* 2007; **30**: 2608–12.

6. Azad N, Emanuele NV, Abraira C *et al.* The effects of intensive glycemic control on neuropathy in the VA cooperative study on type II diabetes mellitus (VACSDM). *J Diabetes Complications* 1999; **13**: 307–13.

7. Oates PJ. Aldose reductase, still a compelling target for diabetic neuropathy. *Curr Drug Targets* 2008; **9**: 14–36.

8. Airey M, Bennett C, Nicolucci A, Williams R. Aldose reductase inhibitors for the prevention and treatment of diabetic peripheral neuropathy. *Cochrane Database Syst Rev* 2000; **2**: CD002182.

9. Toth C, Martinez J, Zochodne DW. RAGE, diabetes, and the nervous system. *Curr Mol Med* 2007; **7**: 766–76.

10. Malik RA, Williamson S, Abbott CA *et al.* Effect of angiotensin-converting enzyme (ACE) inhibitor trandolapril on human diabetic neuropathy: randomised double-blind controlled trial. *Lancet* 1998; **352**: 1978–81.

11. Fried LF, Forrest KY, Ellis D, Chang Y, Silvers N, Orchard TJ. Lipid modulation in insulin-dependent diabetes mellitus: effect on microvascular outcomes. *J Diabetes Complications* 2001; **15**: 113–9.

12. Calcutt NA, Jolivalt CG, Fernyhough P. Growth factors as therapeutics for diabetic neuropathy. *Curr Drug Targets* 2008; **9**: 47–59.

13. Apfel SC, Schwartz S, Adornato BT *et al.* Efficacy and safety of recombinant human nerve growth factor in patients with diabetic polyneuropathy: a randomized controlled trial. *JAMA* 2000; **284**: 2215–21.

14. Wellmer A, Misra VP, Sharief MK, Kopelman PG, Anand P. A double-blind placebo-controlled clinical trial of recombinant human brain-derived neurotrophic factor (rhBDNF) in diabetic polyneuropathy. *J Peripher Nerv Syst* 2001; **6**: 204–10.

15. Sorensen L, Molyneaux L, Yue DK. The relationship among pain, sensory loss, and small nerve fibers in diabetes. *Diabetes Care* 2006; **29**(4): 883–7.

16. Shun CT, Chang YC, Wu HP *et al.* Skin denervation in type 2 diabetes: correlations with diabetic duration and functional impairments. *Brain* 2004; **127**(7): 1593–605.

17. Misawa S, Kuwabara S, Kanai K *et al.* Nodal persistent Na+ currents in human diabetic nerves estimated by the technique of latent addition. *Clin Neurophysiol* 2006; **117**(4): 815–20.

18. Schattschneider J, Scarano M, Binder A *et al.* Modulation of sensitized C-fibers by adrenergic stimulation in human neuropathic pain. *Eur J Pain* 2008; **12**: 517–24.

19. Quattrini C, Harris ND, Malik RA, Tesfaye S. Impaired skin microvascular reactivity in painful diabetic neuropathy. *Diabetes Care* 2007; **30**(3): 655–9.

20. Selvarajah D, Wilkinson ID, Emery CJ *et al.* Early involvement of the spinal cord in diabetic peripheral neuropathy. *Diabetes Care* 2006; **29**: 2664–9.

Chapter 3

Clinical features of diabetic peripheral and autonomic neuropathies

Solomon Tesfaye

Key points

- Diabetic polyneuropathy encompasses a number of neuropathic syndromes, the commonest of which is chronic diabetic peripheral neuropathy (DPN).
- DPN is associated with significant morbidity and mortality.
- Clinical assessment must include a careful history, inquiring about sensory, autonomic, and motor symptoms.
- Other possible causes for neuropathy should be excluded.
- Peripheral neurological examination should include: inspection of the feet and legs, assessment of sensory modalities including the 10 g monofilament test and examination of ankle and knee reflexes.
- Finally footwear should be inspected for poor fit, abnormal wear, and internal pressure areas or foreign bodies.
- Cardiac autonomic neuropathy is a serious complication of diabetes that can result in sudden death.
- Diabetic autonomic neuropathy has many manifestations.

3.1 Introduction

Diabetic polyneuropathy is one of the commonest complications of the diabetes and the commonest form of neuropathy in the Western world. It is not a single entity; it encompasses a number of neuropathic syndromes, the commonest of which is chronic diabetic peripheral neuropathy (DPN), also known as distal symmetrical polyneuropathy (Figure 3.1).

3.2 Classification of diabetic polyneuropathy

A number of classifications for diabetic polyneuropathy have been proposed including one by PK Thomas (1) (Figure 3.1) that subdivides diabetic polyneuropathy into symmetrical and asymmetrical neuropathies. Watkins and Edmonds (2) have suggested an alternative classification based on the natural history of the various syndromes (Box 3.1).

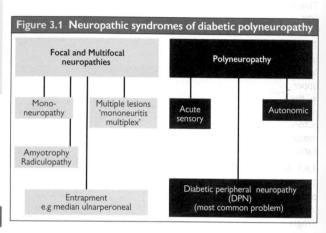

Figure 3.1 Neuropathic syndromes of diabetic polyneuropathy

Focal and Multifocal neuropathies
- Mono-neuropathy
- Amyotrophy Radiculopathy
- Multiple lesions 'mononeuritis multiplex'
- Entrapment e.g median ulnarperoneal

Polyneuropathy
- Acute sensory
- Autonomic
- Diabetic peripheral neuropathy (DPN) (most common problem)

Box 3.1 Classification of diabetic neuropathy based on natural history (2)

1. *Progressive neuropathies.* These are associated with increasing duration of diabetes and with other microvascular complications. Sensory disturbance predominates and autonomic involvement is common. The onset is gradual and there is no recovery.
2. *Reversible neuropathies.* These have an acute onset, often occurring at the presentation of diabetes itself, and are not related to the duration of diabetes or other microvascular complications. There is spontaneous recovery of these acute neuropathies.
3. *Pressure palsies.* Although these are not specific to diabetes only, they tend to occur more frequently in diabetic patients than the general population. There is no association with duration of diabetes or other microvascular complications of diabetes.

3.3 Cardiac consequences of diabetic polyneuropathy

Diabetic polyneuropathy can involve almost every system of the human body, and result in devastating consequences. It is a cause of considerable morbidity and increased mortality. Figure 3.2 summarizes the clinical consequences of diabetic polyneuropathy.

3.4 Diabetic peripheral neuropathy

This is the most common neuropathic syndrome accounting for over 90% of cases and what is meant in clinical practice by the phrase 'diabetic neuropathy' or 'diabetic peripheral neuropathy (DPN)'. There is a 'length-related' pattern of sensory loss, with sensory symptoms starting in the toes and then extending to involve the feet and legs in a stocking distribution. In more severe cases, there may be upper limb involvement, with a similar progression proximally starting in the fingers. Though sub-clinical neuropathy detectable by autonomic function tests is usually present, overtly manifest symptomatic autonomic neuropathy is less common. As the disease advances, clear motor manifestations such as wasting of the small muscles of the hands and limb weakness become apparent.

3.4.1 Symptoms

The main clinical presentation of DPN is sensory loss which the patient may not be aware of, or may be described as 'numbness' or 'dead feeling' of affected limbs. However, some may experience a progressive build-up of unpleasant sensory symptoms including tingling (paraesthesiae); burning pain; shooting pains down the legs; lancinating

19

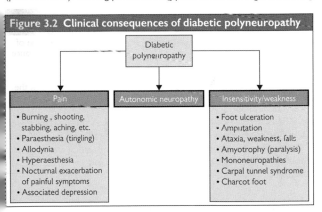

Figure 3.2 Clinical consequences of diabetic polyneuropathy

Diabetic polyneuropathy

Pain	Autonomic neuropathy	Insensitivity/weakness
• Burning , shooting, stabbing, aching, etc.		• Foot ulceration
• Paraesthesia (tingling)		• Amputation
• Allodynia		• Ataxia, weakness, falls
• Hyperaesthesia		• Amyotrophy (paralysis)
• Nocturnal exacerbation of painful symptoms		• Mononeuropathies
• Associated depression		• Carpal tunnel syndrome
		• Charcot foot

pains; contact pain often with daytime clothes and bed clothes (allodynia); pain on walking often described as walking barefoot on 'broken glass', 'hot sand', 'pebbles', 'cotton wool'; sensations of heat or cold in the feet; persistent achy feeling in the feet and cramp-like sensations in the legs. For a full description of painful DPN including acute sensory (painful) neuropathies, refer to Chapter 5.

Autonomic neuropathy (AN) has varied presentations depending on the affected system (Figure 3.2). Clinical consultation must ascertain if there are cardiovascular symptoms (dizziness or fainting on standing, exercise intolerance, etc.), upper gastrointestinal symptoms (bloating, nausea, vomiting, glycaemic swings associated with gastroparesis, anorexia, weight loss, etc.), lower gastrointestinal symptoms (diarrhoea, faecal incontinence, constipation), erectile dysfunction, bladder problems (urinary retention or incontinence), excessive sweating often associated with eating (gustatory sweating), pupillary reflex abnormalities in response to light, and so on.

It is important to appreciate that many patients with DPN may not have any of the above sensory or autonomic symptoms, and their first presentation may be with a foot ulcer (3). This underpins the need for carefully examining and screening the feet of all diabetic people in order to identify those at risk of developing foot ulceration (4). An intriguing feature of the neuropathic foot is that both numbness and pain may occur, the so-called 'painful, painless' leg (5). It is indeed a paradox that the patient with a large foot ulcer may also have severe neuropathic pain (5). In those with advanced neuropathy, there may be sensory ataxia resulting in unsteadiness on walking and falls particularly if there is associated visual impairment due to retinopathy.

3.4.2 **Signs**

Neuropathy is usually easily detected by simple clinical examination. Shoes and socks should be removed and the feet examined at least annually (during annual review) and more often if neuropathy is present. The most common presenting abnormality is a reduction or absence of vibration sense in the toes. As the disease progresses, there is sensory loss in a 'stocking' and sometimes in a 'glove' distribution involving all modalities (including light touch, pinprick sensation as well as cold and heat sensations) (Figure 3.3). When there is severe sensory loss, proprioception may also be impaired (loss of position sense), leading to a positive Romberg's sign. Ankle tendon reflexes are lost and with more advanced neuropathy, knee reflexes are reduced or absent. The 10 g monofilament test, which is quick and easy to perform by the bedside, is reduced or absent. An abnormal test is predictive of future development of foot ulceration (Table 3.1).

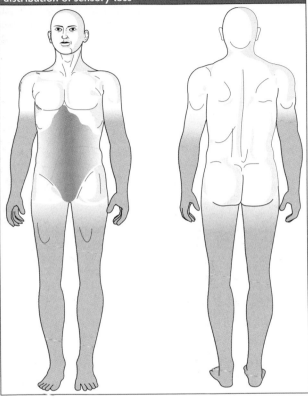

Figure 3.3 DPN presenting with a glove and stocking distribution of sensory loss

Muscle strength is usually normal early during the course of the disease. With progressive disease there is significant generalized muscular wasting, particularly in the small muscles of the hands and feet. The fine movements of fingers would then be affected, and there is difficulty in handling small objects. The clawing of the toes is believed to be due to unopposed (because of wasting of the small muscles of the foot) pulling of the long extensor and flexor tendons. This results in elevated plantar pressure points at the metatarsal heads that are prone to callus formation and foot ulceration (4). Foot deformities such as a bunion and Charcot neuroarthropathy can form the focus of ulceration (6). Inappropriate footwear is the most

Table 3.1 Summary of clinical assessment for DPN	
History	Signs
• Sensory symptoms	Inspection
• Motor symptoms	Reflexes
• Assessment of disability	Sensory
• Exclude other causes of neuropathy	• Vibration
	• Light touch
	• Pinprick
	• 10g Monofilament
	Assess footwear

common form of trauma to the neuropathic foot and thus a thorough assessment should also include examination of shoes for poor fit, abnormal wear, and internal pressure areas or foreign bodies (4) (Table 3.1).

AN affecting the feet can cause a reduction in sweating and consequently dry skin that is likely to crack easily, predisposing the patient to the risk of infection (4). The 'purely' neuropathic foot is also warm due to artero-venous shunting first described by Ward (7). This results in the distension of foot veins that fail to collapse even when the foot is elevated. It is not unusual to observe a gangrenous toe in a foot that has bounding arterial pulses, as there is impairment of the nutritive capillary circulation due to arterio-venous shunting. The oxygen tension of the blood in these foot veins is typically raised (8). The increasing blood flow brought about by AN can sometimes result in neuropathic oedema, which is resistant to treatment with diuretics but may respond to treatment with ephedrine (9).

3.5 **Natural history of DPN**

The natural history of DPN remains poorly understood because of lack of well-designed prospective studies. One study (10) reported that neuropathic symptoms remain or get worse over a 5-year period in patients with DPN. A major drawback of this study was that it involved highly selected patients from a hospital base. Another study reported improvements in painful symptoms with worsening of quantitative measures of nerve function over 3½ years (11). At follow-up, 3½ years later, one-third of the 50 patients had died or were lost to follow-up. Clearly, this is also a major drawback. There was symptomatic improvement in painful neuropathy in the majority of the remaining patients. It should be noted that many of the subjects were being treated with pain-relieving drugs that may also have influenced the findings. Despite symptomatic improvement, small fibre function deteriorated significantly.

3.6 **Differential diagnosis of DPN**

DPN presents in a similar way to neuropathies of other causes, and thus the physician needs to carefully exclude other common causes before attributing the neuropathy to diabetes (Box 3.2). Absence of other complications of diabetes, rapid weight loss, excessive alcohol intake, and other atypical features in either the history or clinical examination, should alert the physician to search for other causes of neuropathy.

3.7 **Autonomic neuropathy**

Abnormalities of autonomic function are very common in subjects with long-standing diabetes; however, clinically significant autonomic dysfunction is uncommon. Several systems can be affected (Box 3.3). Box 3.4 shows typical questions aimed at evaluating the presence of AN. AN has a gradual onset and is slowly progressive. The prevalence of diabetic autonomic neuropathy depends on the type of population studied, and a number of tests of autonomic function employed.

Box 3.2 **Differential diagnosis of DPN**

Metabolic
- Diabetes
- Amyloidosis
- Uraemia
- Myxoedema
- Porphyria
- Vitamin deficiency (thiamine, B12, B6, pyridoxine)

Drugs and chemicals
- Alcohol
- Cytotoxic drugs, e.g. vincristine, chlorambucil
- Nitrofurantoin
- Isoniazid

Neoplastic disorders
- Bronchial or gastric carcinoma

Lymphoma

Infective or inflammatory
- Leprosy
- Guillain–Barre syndrome
- Lyme borreliosis
- Chronic inflammatory demyelinating polyneuropathy
- Polyarteritis nodosa

Genetic

Charcot-Marie-Tooth disease
- Hereditary sensory neuropathies

CHAPTER 3 C

autonomic neuropathy causes postural hypotension, ...heral blood flow, and may be a cause of sudden death.

...al features ... *hypotension*

...now generally accepted that a fall in systolic blood pressure (BP) of >20 mmHg is considered abnormal. Coincidental treatment with tricyclic antidepressants for neuropathic pain, and diuretics may exacerbate postural hypotension, the chief symptom of which is dizziness on standing. The symptoms of postural hypotension can be disabling for some patients who may not be able to walk for more

---

Box 3.3 Clinical manifestations of diabetic autonomic neuropathy

- Cardiovascular
  - Resting tachycardia, orthostasis, loss of beat to beat variation, systolic and diastolic dysfunction, cardiac denervation
  - Failure of hypoxia-induced respiratory drive
  - Obstructive sleep apnoea
- Gastrointestinal
  - Gastroparesis, constipation, diarrhoea
- Genitourinary
  - Erectile dysfunction incontinence, vaginal dryness
- Neurovascular
  - Dry skin, cold or hot feet due to poor or excessive blood flow, gustatory sweating, hyperhidrosis; pupilomotor dysfunction
- Metabolic
  - Hypoglycaemia unawareness, severe hypoglycaemia, glycaemic swing

---

Box 3.4 Symptom evaluation for diabetic autonomic neuropathy

- Do you faint when you stand up?
- Do you have problems with erections?
- Do you have trouble controlling your bladder?
- Do you have diarrhoea?
- Do you have constipation?
- How is your appetite?
- Do you get full quickly or feel bloated?
- Do you vomit after eating?
- Do you have blood glucose swings?
- Do you sweat when you eat?
- Do you sweat when it's not hot?
- Do lights from oncoming cars bother your eyes when driving at night?
- Do you have hypoglycaemia unawareness?

a few minutes. In clinical practice, the severity of dizziness does
correlate with the postural drop in BP. There is increased mor-
lity in subjects with postural hypotension, although the reasons for
his are not fully clear. The management of subjects with postural
hypotension is discussed in Chapter 6.

3.7.1.2 Cardiovascular autonomic function tests

Box 3.5 shows indications for cardiovascular autonomic testing and
Table 3.2 shows the various tests of parasympathetic and sympathetic
function. Five cardiovascular autonomic function tests are now widely
used for the assessment of autonomic function in clinical practice.
These tests are non-invasive, and do not require sophisticated equip-
ment (all that is required is an electrocardiogram machine, an aneroid
pressure gauge attached to a mouthpiece, a hand grip dynamometer,
and sphygmomanometer). Table 3.3 shows reference list for cardiovascular autonomic function test.

Box 3.5 Indications for cardiovascular autonomic testing

- Orthostatic hypotension
- Dizziness and syncope
- Unexplained tachycardia
- Presence of other organ manifestations of AN
  - Erectile dysfunction, gastroparesis
- Pre-operative risk assessment

Table 3.2 Tests of autonomic function

Parasympathetic	Sympathetic
• Resting heart rate	• Resting heart rate
• Beat to beat variation with deep breathing (E:I ratio)	• Spectral analysis of heart rate variation, low frequency power (LFP <0.14 Hz)
• 30:15 heart rate ratio with standing	• Orthostasis BP
• Valsalva ratio	• Hand grip BP
• Spectral analysis of heart rate variation, high frequency power (HFP 0.15–0.40 Hz)	• Cold pressor response
	• Sympathetic skin galvanic response (cholinergic)
	• Sudorimetry (cholinergic)
	• Cutaneous blood flow (peptidergic)

Sympathetic/parasympathetic balance = LFP/HFP.

Table 3.3 Reference values for cardiovascular function tests

	Normal	Borderline	Abnormal
Heart rate tests Heart rate response to standing up (30:15 ratio)	>1.04	1.01–1.03	<1.00
Heart rate response to deep breathing (maximum minus minimum heart rate)	>15 beats/min	11–14 beats/min	<10 beats/min
Heart rate response to Valsalva manoeuvre (Valsalva ratio)	>1.21	—	<1.20
BP tests BP response to standing up (fall in systolic BP)	<10 mmHg	11–29 mmHg	>30 mmHg
BP response to sustained handgrip (increase in diastolic BP)	>16 mmHg	11–15 mmHg	<10 mmHg

Adapted from Ewing DJ, Martyn CN, Young RJ, Clarke BF (1985). The value of cardiovascular autonomic function tests: ten years experience in diabetes. *Diabetes Care,* **8**: 491–8.

3.8 Conclusions

- Diabetic polyneuropathy is not a single entity but encompasses a number of neuropathic syndromes, the commonest of which is DPN.
- DPN is a cause of considerable morbidity and increased mortality.
- Clinical assessment must include a careful history, inquiring about sensory, autonomic, and motor symptoms, as well assessing disability as a result of DPN. Other causes for neuropathy should be excluded. Peripheral neurological examination should include: inspection of the feet and legs, assessment of sensory modalities including the 10 g monofilament test, and examination of ankle and knee reflexes.
- Finally, footwear should be inspected for poor fit, abnormal wear, and internal pressure areas or foreign bodies.
- Cardiovascular autonomic neuropathy is a serious complication of diabetes that may result in troublesome postural hypotension, exercise intolerance, and sudden death.
- Standard bedside cardiovascular autonomic function tests are available for the assessment of autonomic function in clinical practice.

References

1. Thomas PK. Metabolic neuropathy. *J Roy Coll Phys (Lond)* 1973; **7**: 154.

2. Watkins PJ, Edmonds ME. Clinical features of diabetic neuropathy. In *Textbook of Diabetes*, Vol. 2. Pickup J, Williams G (Eds.). 1997; pp. 50.1–50.20.

3. Tesfaye S. Diabetic neuropathy: achieving best practice. *Br J Vasc Dis* 2003; **3**: 112–7.

4. Boulton AJM, Kirsner RS, Viliekyte L. Neuropathic diabetic foot ulcers. *N Engl J Med* 2004; **351**: 48–55.

5. Ward JD. The diabetic leg. *Diabetologia* 1982; **22**: 141–7.

6. Rajbhandari SM, Jenkins R, Davies C, Tesfaye S. Charcot neuroarthropathy in diabetes mellitus. *Diabetologia* 2002; **45**: 1085–96.

7. Ward JD, Simms JM, Knight G, Boulton AJM, Sandler DA. Venous distension in the diabetic neuropathic foot (physical sign of arterio-venous shunting). *J Roy Soc Med* 1983; **76**: 1011–4.

8. Boulton AJM, Scarpello JHB, Ward JD. Venous oxygenation in the diabetic neuropathic foot: evidence of arterial venous shunting? *Diabetologia* 1982; **22**: 6–8.

9. Edmonds ME, Archer AG, Watkins PJ. Ephedrine: a new treatment for diabetic neuropathic oedema. *Lancet* 1983; **i**: 548–51.

10. Boulton AJM, Armstrong WD, Scarpello JHB, Ward JD. The natural history of painful diabetic neuropathy—a 4 year study. *Postgrad Med J* 1983; **59**: 556–9.

11. Benbow SJ, Chan AW, Bowsher D, McFarlane IA, Williams G. A prospective study of painful symptoms, small fibre function and peripheral vascular disease in chronic painful diabetic neuropathy. *Diabet Med* 1994; **11**: 17–21.

12. Ewing DJ, Martyn CN, Young RJ, Clarke BF. The value of cardiovascular autonomic function tests: ten years experience in diabetes. *Diabetes Care* 1985; **8**: 491–8.

Chapter 4

Diagnosis of diabetic peripheral neuropathy— clinical practice and research

Andrew J M Boulton

Key points

- Diabetic peripheral neuropathy (DPN) is a clinical diagnosis in day-to-day practice; it is a diagnosis of exclusion of other causes and a simple history and clinical examination are the essential components.
- As up to 50% of patients may be asymptomatic the diagnosis cannot be made on history alone.
- For clinical research, the diagnosis of DPN requires at least two tests in addition to the clinical history and examination: these normally comprise quantitative sensory testing (QST) and electrophysiology (EP).
- Although EP remains the gold standard for clinical research in DPN, promising new techniques include skin biopsy and confocal corneal microscopy (CCM).
- Peripheral sympathetic autonomic neuropathy can lead to a warm, dry foot in the absence of peripheral vascular disease. For clinical research, tests such as galvanic skin resistance or the newer Neuropad® may be used.

4.1 Introduction

The annual review, where all patients with diabetes should be screened for evidence of microvascular complications on an annual basis, has become a keystone in diabetes management in western countries. An important component of the annual review is screening for diabetic neuropathy (DPN) in the lower limbs. For the rest of this chapter, the term DPN will refer to distal symmetrical somatic polyneuropathy; mention will also be made of diabetic peripheral autonomic neuropathy (DPAN) which is also commonly found in the lower limbs.

The diagnosis of DPN will be considered under three main headings:

1. In primary care, screening of the lower limbs is most important to answer the question 'Is this patient at risk of insensitive foot ulceration or injury as a consequence of sensory loss?'

2. Screening for DPN in clinical practice may be used to diagnose early neuropathy or to help diagnose the aetiology of pain in a patient complaining of neuropathic symptomatology in the lower limbs.

3. The diagnosis of the presence or absence of DPN for clinical research purposes needs a much more detailed assessment and in addition to history and examination requires other tests such as quantitative sensory testing (QST) and electrophysiology (EP).

The chapter will therefore be divided into three sections, describing the approach to the diagnosis of neuropathy for each of the above situations.

4.2 Diagnosis of DPN in the annual review— is this patient at risk of foot ulceration?

The two key components of the assessment at the annual review are history and examination of the lower limb (1). Key features in the history refer to past or present reporting of neuropathic symptoms or insensitive injury. When taking the history, it is essential to document patients' exact descriptions of symptoms avoiding leading the questions. Neuropathic pain is difficult to describe because it is unfamiliar to the patient (in contrast with nociceptive pain). Some typical symptoms and signs of DPN are listed in Table 4.1. It must be remembered that

Table 4.1 Stages, symptoms, and signs of DPN	
State of neuropathy	Characteristics
No neuropathy	
Clinical neuropathy	Burning, shooting, stabbing pain
• Chronic painful	• Uncomfortable 'electrical' sensations: numbness, paraesthesias, nocturnal exacerbation. Absent sensation to several modalities; reduced/absent ankle reflexes
• Acute painful	• Severe symptoms as above: may follow episode of glycaemic instability; few signs
• Painless	• Numbness/deadness of feet or no symptoms. Reduced/absent sensation. Absent ankle reflexes
• Late complications	• Foot lesions; callus; neuropathic deformity; non-traumatic amputation
Abridged from Boulton et al. (2).	

p to half of those at risk of insensitive foot ulceration may have no history of neuropathic symptoms and another sizeable minority might have a history of typical symptoms some years prior to the examination which have been subsequently resolved.

Examination should include an assessment of the integrity of the peripheral nervous system:

- Inspection of both feet: skin status, sweating (absence of sweating is indication of DPAN), ulceration, calluses, deformity, muscle wasting
- Assessment of peripheral sensation (3; 4):
    - Peripheral sensation–vibration (128 Hz Tuning Fork over apex of great toe
    - Pain sensation over distal hallux using pin or neurotip
    - Hot/cold differentiation using hot/cold rods (5)
    - Ankle reflexes
- Simple bedside tests: 10 g monofilaments (6). The ability to perceive pressure using a 10 g monofilament is a useful screening test for sensory loss and risk of foot ulceration. The recent American Diabetes Association (ADA) recommendations (4) suggest testing at four sites on each foot: first, third, and fifth meta-tarsal heads and plantar surface of distal hallux. Failure to detect 10 g pressure when the monofilament buckles at any site on either foot suggests risk of insensitive injury.

If available, vibration perception threshold (VPT) can be tested over the hallux using a biothesiometer (Horwell, Nottingham, UK) (5).

The recent ADA guidelines suggest that any two of the above tests/ examinations can be used to identify the foot at risk of ulceration. A simple composite score of sensory and reflex deficit, the modified neuropathy disability score, has been shown to be highly predictive of subsequent foot ulceration (3); this is a simple score of three sensory modalities over the hallux (vibration, pain, and hot/cold differentiation) together with the ankle reflexes. The 10 g monofilaments are widely used in screening for the high risk foot; however, as highlighted by Booth and Young (7), some monofilaments may not be accurate at assessing pressure at 10 g. Caution should therefore be exercised when selecting which monofilament to use.

4.3 Clinical practice—are these symptoms due to DPN?

As noted by Ziegler in Chapter 1, the DPN is a common complication of diabetes and up to 50% of patients with this condition will experience symptoms, although not all will require specific therapies. This chapter is not referring to other types of symptomatic neuropathy which are less commonly seen in diabetes and might include the mononeuropathies, proximal motor neuropathy (or amyotrophy) or the truncal neuropathies (5). Whereas the symptoms experienced by patients with both acute and chronic DPN are similar, they tend to be of much more rapid onset and severe in those with acute DPN; typically, this form of neuropathy occurs after a period of poor glycaemic control, such as diabetic ketoacidosis, or even after starting oral hypoglycaemic agents or insulin. In contrast, the symptoms of chronic DPN are of gradual or insidious onset and tend to be associated with signs of sensory loss and reduced or absent ankle reflexes (Table 4.1). The history and clinical examination are usually strongly suggestive of the diagnosis of chronic DPN; however, there are no specific tests that will identify the neuropathy as secondary to diabetes. The diagnosis is therefore one of exclusion and other conditions that may masquerade as a peripheral neuropathy in a patient with diabetes include underlying malignancy, hypothfoidism, vitamin B12 deficiency, human immunodeficiency virus (HIV), drug therapies (especially for malignant diseases), toxin exposure, and paraproteinaemia. Moreover, the typical DPN is almost invariably symmetrical in a predominantly stocking distribution. There are a number of features that would be atypical of DPN and these are listed in Box 4.1 and should warrant referral to a neurologist.

In clinical practice, the diagnosis is generally made by the history and examination together with a number of normal tests excluding other conditions listed earlier. Occasionally, the diagnosis might prove difficult and referral for QST and/or electrophysiological investigation is therefore indicated (see below).

The differentiation of neuropathic pain from that induced by peripheral vascular disease is generally not a clinical challenge. Occasionally, however, neuropathic pain may masquerade as 'atypical' claudication. It should be remembered that classical intermittent claudication is a consequence of proximal arterial disease and is characterized by pain in the muscles of the leg induced by exercise and relieved by rest within minutes without change of position. Atypical claudication usually requires some change of position to relieve the pain such as leaning forward or sitting down. Such symptoms might suggest 'neurogenic' claudication and spinal investigation to exclude spinal stenosis are indicated prior to labelling this 'atypical claudication' as a manifestation of diabetic peripheral neuropathy.

Box 4.1 Findings that might precipitate neurology referral

- Asymmetrical symptoms or signs
- Predominant motor signs
- Marked muscle wasting
- Rapid progression
- Neck or back pain
- Family history of neuropathy

4.4 **Diagnosis of DPN for clinical research studies**

The primary aim of the previous two sections was the correct identification of those patients who are at risk of insensitive foot injury and confirm that those who experience neuropathic symptoms were suffering from DPN. In contrast, the focus of this section will not only be in showing that the diagnosis of DPN is correct for clinical research studies, but also in the quantification of the neurological deficit. In clinical research studies of potential new agents for the management of diabetic neuropathy, each subject should be entered into the trial at a well-defined point in the natural history of DPN; the methods employed in obtaining these data must therefore have high levels of reproducibility, sensitivity, and specificity for both the diagnosis of DPN and in assessing its progress.

4.4.1 **Clinical assessment**

The clinical assessment, that is, measurement of symptoms and signs, is just as important in clinical research as it is in clinical examination. Assessment of symptoms, for example, is crucial in the assessment of new therapies for the relief of pain in patients with DPN. Neuropathic symptoms are often assessed using a visual analogue scale such as the 10-cm graphic rating scale (5). A number of composite scores for assessing clinical end points such as symptoms and signs have been developed and these range from the very simple modified neuropathy symptom score and neuropathy disability score (5) to the more complex and well-validated scales many of which have been developed by Grant *et al.* (8). The Neuropathy Symptom and Change (NSC) score is one such example and comprises a set of 38 questions that assess the severity and change of symptoms of DPN. A scoring system for neurological deficits (signs) that focuses on the lower limb, known as the neuropathy impairment score in the lower limbs (NIS-LL), is frequently used in longitudinal clinical studies (9).

4.4.2 **Quantitative sensory testing**

The hallmark of DPN is the progressive loss or change in sensation in the lower limbs. Measures of QST can identify which sensory modalities are affected as well as measuring the magnitude of that deficit. In previous studies of DPN, assessment of vibration, thermal and pain thresholds have proven valuable in the detection of sub-clinical neuropathy as well as tracking progression of neuropathy in large cohorts. QST measures have also played a pivotal role in primary efficacy end point in a series of large multicentre trials. As with all tests, QST has well-documented strengths and weaknesses; strengths include the ability to assess multiple modalities, the use of well-established psychophysical procedures as well as the capacity to measure function over a wide range of intensities. The major limitation of QST is that no matter how sophisticated the instrument used, it is only a semi-quantitative measure which relies upon patient feedback and therefore will be affected by the subject's attention, motivation, and co-operation.

A number of instruments are available to test VPT. These range from the simple measures such as the biothesiometer, comprising a hand-held probe the vibration of which can be controlled by a simple dial. Using this simple machine, loss of vibration perception has been shown to be a strong predictor of subsequent ulceration (5). Much more sophisticated devices such as the computer-aided sensory examination (CASE) have been used in clinical trials of new putative agents to slow the progression of diabetic neuropathy.

Thermal thresholds are also frequently measured in clinical trials and separate cold and warm thermoreceptors have been identified. Thermal energy is conducted in small nerve fibres and high-intensity stimulation of these receptors (especially those sensitive to warming) can be used to assess heat-pain thresholds. The CASE system in addition to measuring vibration can also be used to assess thermal thresholds: for both vibration and thermal, precise and consistent stimuli are administered in a controlled manner during testing (1).

4.4.3 **Electrophysiology**

Nerve conduction studies (NCS) have for many years been the gold standard in the measurement of neuropathy in clinical trials. As well as correlating well with underlying structural changes, NCS can be measured without requiring any input from the patient and therefore highly reproducible with low coefficient of variation. However, NCS are not sensitive to small fibre changes. In clinical trials, tests of both sensory and motor nerves are typically used often using the median and ulnar nerve in the upper limb and the sural and peroneal nerves in the lower limbs. Despite the fact that abnormalities of NCS are typically found in cases of DPN, this cannot be used as a diagnostic test as it simply identifies that an abnormality is present but cannot distinguish whether this is due to diabetes or other causes.

4.4.4 **Nerve biopsy**

In the past, some studies have included biopsies of the sural nerve to enable detailed morphological analysis to be undertaken. However, this is an invasive procedure and is now rarely used in clinical trials as repeat biopsies are necessary.

The selection of appropriate surrogate or actual end points in clinical trials of new agents of DPN was recently covered in an editorial (10). It appears that the natural progression of DPN is actually much slower than previously believed, thus some of the traditional end points such as QST and NCS discussed earlier might not be appropriate, at least alone, in future trials of potential new treatments.

Two more recently developed techniques for assessing peripheral nerve function might therefore be useful surrogate end points for future clinical trials. The first of these is the assessment of intra-epidermal nerve fibres taken from punch skin biopsies. Although invasive, this investigation is minimally so and has been used in a few studies to monitor progress. The assessment of these fibres is particularly useful for studies of small fibre neurological dysfunction in diabetes.

Similarly, the non-invasive corneal confocal microscopy has been developed and might be an ideal technique that can be repeatedly performed to assess progression of DPN in future clinical trials (11). This study showed that changes in corneal nerve fibres parallel those seen in diabetic neuropathy assessed in the lower limbs. The advantage of this technique is that it is completely non-invasive.

4.5 **Diabetic peripheral autonomic neuropathy**

The diagnosis of DPAN is often assumed in those with DPN because of the finding of a warm foot with dry skin and often distended dorsal foot veins. These are all signs of peripheral sympathetic dysfunction, and the lack of sweating is very common in the foot at risk of insensitive ulceration. Although has rarely been quantified in the past, the recent development of an indicator plaster which when applied to the skin changes colour from blue to pink if sweating is present, raising the possibility of the use of a simple test to diagnose the at risk foot. A recent study (12) showed that abnormalities assessed by this Neuropad® correlated well with standard measures of both somatic and autonomic dysfunction. Similarly, another recent study (13) has even suggested that this simple test might be administered by patients at home for self-testing in the identification of those at risk of insensitive ulceration.

4.6 **Conclusion**

In summary, the diagnosis of DPN for clinical practice is a clinical one in which the history and examination are crucial parts and the exclusion of non-diabetic causes by appropriate investigations usually confirms the cause to be diabetes. For clinical trials, other more precise investigations are essential to quantify and measure neurological deficit. Clinical guidelines for the diagnosis and outpatient management of diabetic peripheral neuropathy have been published (2), and a more recent physician statement by the ADA (14) describes the approach to the diagnosis and management of DPN.

References

1. Scott LV, Tesfaye S. Measurement of somatic neuropathy for clinical practice and clinical trials. *Curr Diab Rep* 2001; **1**: 208–15.

2. Boulton AJ, Gries FA, Jervell JA. Guidelines for the diagnosis and outpatient management of diabetic peripheral neuropathy. *Diabet Med* 1998; **15**: 508–14.

3. Abbott CA, Carrington AL, Ashe H et al. The North-West Diabetes Foot Care Study: incidence of, and risk factors for, new diabetic foot ulceration in a community-based patient cohort. *Diabet Med* 2002; **19**: 377–384.

4. Boulton AJM, Armstrong DG, Albert SF et al. Comprehensive foot exam and risk assessment: a report of the American Diabetes Association task force on foot care. *Diabetes Care* 2008; **31**: 1679–85.

5. Boulton AJ, Malik RA, Arezzo JC, Sosenko JM. Diabetic somatic neuropathies. *Diabetes Care* 2004; **27**: 1458–86.

6. Mayfield JE, Sugarman JR. The use of Semmes–Weinstein monofilaments and other tests for preventing foot ulceration and amputation in people with diabetes. *J Fam Pract* 2000; **49** (Suppl 1): 517–29.

7. Booth J, Young MJ. Differences in the performance of commercially available 10-g monofilaments. *Diabetes Care* 2000; **23**: 984–8.

8. Grant IA, O'Brien P, Dyck PJ. Neuropathy tests and normative results. In *Diabetic Neuropathy*, 2nd edition. Duck PJ, Thomas PK, Eds. WB Saunders, Philadelphia 1999; pp. 124–40.

9. Bril V. NIS-LL the primary measurement scale for clinical trial endpoints in diabetic peripheral neuropathy. *Eur Neurol* 1999; **41** (Suppl 1): 8–13.

10. Boulton AJM. Whither clinical research in diabetic sensorimotor peripheral neuropathy? Problems of end point selection for clinical trials. *Diabetes Care* 2007; **30**: 2752–3.

11. Malik RA, Kallinikos P, Abbott CA et al. Corneal confocal microscopy: a non-invasive surrogate of nerve fibre damage and repair in diabetic patients. *Diabetologia* 2003; **46**: 683–8.

12. Quattrini C, Jeziorska M, Tavakoli M et al. The Neuropad® test: a visual indicator test for human diabetic neuropathy. *Diabetologia* 2008; **51**: 1046–50.

13. Tentolouris N, Archtsidis V, Marinou K, Katsilambros N. Evaluation of the self-administered indicator plaster Neuropad® for the diagnosis of neuropathy in diabetes. *Diabetes Care* 2008; **31**: 236–7.

14. Boulton AJ, Vinik AI, Arezzo JC et al. Diabetic neuropathies: a statement by the American Diabetes Association. *Diabetes Care* 2005; **28**: 956–62.

Chapter 5

Assessment and management of painful diabetic peripheral neuropathy

Solomon Tesfaye

Key points

- Painful diabetic peripheral neuropathy (DPN) is common and can be distressing. However, despite this, it continues to be under-diagnosed and under-treated.
- The minimum requirements for diagnosis of painful DPN are assessment of symptoms and neurological examination, with shoes and sock removed. Bilateral sensory impairment is almost always present.
- Painful diabetic neuropathy is characterized by burning, shooting, or stabbing pain in the extremities. Pain may be spontaneous or evoked.
- Optimization of cardiovascular risk factors and improved glycaemic control are important.
- First-line therapies for painful DPN are tricyclic antidepressants (TCA), serotonin noradrenaline reuptake inhibitors (SNRIs) (such as duloxetine), or anticonvulsants (such as pregabalin or gabapentin), taking into account patients' co-morbidities and cost.
- Combination therapy may be useful although the evidence base is relatively poor.

37

5.1 Painful Diabetic Peripheral Neuropathy

Diabetic peripheral neuropathy (DPN) commonly manifests with sensory loss in stocking and glove distribution that [1] the patient may be aware of described as 'numbness' or 'dead feeling', [2] the patient may not be aware of sometimes resulting in a first presentation of a foot ulcer, and [3] may paradoxically occur in conjunction with painful symptoms in the lower limbs. Approximately one-third of patients with DPN present with painful symptoms affecting the feet and legs, and in advanced cases the upper limbs. Pain is the most distressir symptom of DPN and the main reason for seeking medical attention.

5.2 **Epidemiology**

There are only very few, well-designed studies looking at the prevalence of painful DPN. These report a prevalence rate of 10–26% amongst diabetic patients, reflecting differing criteria used to define neuropathic pain (1). In the EURODIAB prospective study, nearly a quarter of Type 1 patients developed new onset painful DPN over a 7-year period (1). Therefore, painful diabetic neuropathy is a common clinically challenging problem.

5.3 **Clinical features**

Patients with DPN present with slowly progressive sensory loss affecting the lower limbs. Typically, sensory symptoms, if present, will start in the toes and over many years progress to involve the legs, in a stocking distribution. Once the neuropathy is well established in the lower limbs, the upper limbs may be affected. Patients with painful DPN may experience a progressive build-up of unpleasant sensory symptoms including burning pain; shooting pains (like 'electric shock') down the legs; lancinating pain (also likened as 'stabbing' or 'knife-like'); contact pain (allodynia) often with daytime and bed clothes; tingling ('pins and needles', 'prickling', or paraesthesiae); pain on walking often described as walking barefoot on 'marbles', 'hot sand', and so on; sensations of heat or cold in the feet; persistent achy feeling in the feet and cramp-like sensations in the legs. Some may have unusual sensations that are described as 'tightly wrapped feeling of feet', and so on (Box 5.1). There is a large spectrum of severity of these symptoms, with some having only minor complaints such as tingling in one or two toes, whilst others may be affected with more disabling pain that fails to respond standard treatments.

Box 5.1 Symptoms of DPN

Sensory symptoms
- Numbness (dead feeling)
- Paraesthesia (tingling or 'pins and needles')
- Pain (burning, stabbing, shooting, deep aching)
- Unusual sensations ('tightly wrapped' feeling of feet/legs, 'walking on cotton wool', etc.)
- Allodynia (pain evoked by a non-painful stimulus)
- Inability to identify objects in hands

Motor symptoms
- Weakness, e.g. difficulty climbing stairs
- Difficulty lifting/handling small objects

Painful diabetic neuropathy is characteristically more severe at night, and often prevents sleep (2). Affected patients may be in a constant state of tiredness because of sleep deprivation (2). The constant, unremitting pain may also result in depression (2). Pain also has an impact on work and social life. Some of the worst affected patients are unable to maintain full employment. Severe painful neuropathy can occasionally cause marked reduction in exercise threshold thus interfering with daily activities (2).

5.4 **Acute painful neuropathies**

Painful DPN occasionally has an acute onset, with severe painful symptoms emerging within weeks. Patients may present within the context of [1] very poor blood glucose control or after ketoacidosis (usually in Type 1 patients known as 'acute painful neuropathy of poor glycaemic control') or [2] after initiation of glucose-lowering treatment with either insulin or oral agents ('acute painful neuropathy of rapid glycaemic control') (3). These acute syndromes are relatively rare compared to the chronic painful neuropathy associated with DPN, and cause a rapid build-up of painful symptoms within weeks leading to persistent lower limb burning pain and allodynia. There is nocturnal exacerbation of symptoms and depression is a common feature (3). There may also be significant weight loss. Peripheral neurological examination is often unremarkable with either no or mild sensory loss. There are no motor signs. The prognosis in acute painful neuropathies is good with complete resolution of symptoms within a year (3).

5.5 **Assessment of painful diabetic neuropathy**

5.5.1 **History**

The assessment and management of neuropathic pain continues to pose considerable challenge to clinicians (4).

5.5.1.1 *Empathic approach*

Some of the badly affected patients with painful DPN often attend clinic accompanied by family members or relatives and the first thing to do is to get out of chair and invite them into the room and make them feel welcome. The second thing to do is to actually look them in the eye and to show them an empathic face, to say that you understand how they feel, that you know something about it, and that you may be able to help them with certain medications or advice. Many feel terribly misunderstood because there is nothing abnormal to see. They may not even have an ulcer or another obvious problem.

They may also feel that family members or other people do not really fully appreciate their predicament. When they see that the health-care professional does empathize and understand how they feel, the first thing that you will notice is a change in their body language. They become less tense and sit down in a more relaxed fashion. Health-care professionals should not only indicate to them that they are well aware of what they can do to manage their pain, but also try to imagine their pain, and show empathy. Some who may have the appropriate knowledge of managing neuropathic pain may unfortunately be dismissive to the emotional component of the sufferer's pain.

The consultation will uncover that the more severely affected patients may present with a variety of emotions. Some patients feel anxious that their pain will result in amputation. Such a false assumption must be dismissed authoritatively and this can be therapeutic in itself. Others may feel very depressed because of the unremitting pain and this has to be effectively treated. Some may feel intensely angry as this is yet another complication of diabetes on top of the retinopathy, kidney failure, and so on. Many feel very guilty that years of poor control have led to their predicament but they have to be encouraged to look forwards with hope and not backwards. Thus, an empathic approach with a multidisciplinary support is crucial as the psychological impact of painful DPN is considerable (4). The whole team must also speak with same voice. Conflicting information can be extremely counter-productive.

5.5.1.2 *Assessment of symptoms*
A careful history is required to establish that the pain is neuropathic in nature (Box 5.1). Does the patient have typical painful symptoms such as burning, shooting, lancinating, or deep aching pains? Is there allodynia (pain produced by normally non-painful stimulus such as bed cloths)? These symptoms should normally affect the legs in symmetrical fashion. Unilateral leg pain should arouse a suspicion that the pain may be due to lumbar-sacral nerve root compression, or some other pathology.

The quality and severity of neuropathic pain should be assessed preferably using a suitable pain rating scale (e.g. visual analogue scale or numeric rating scale), so that response to treatment may be evaluated. These scales are quick and easy to perform within a context of a busy clinic.

5.5.2 **Clinical examination**
In over 90% of patients, diagnosis of DPN can be made by bedside peripheral neurological/vascular examination (Chapters 3 and 4). Examination will also exclude other possible causes of leg pain such as peripheral vascular disease, prolapsed intervertebral discs, spinal-canal stenosis, and corda aquina lesions. Occasionally, for example, where clinical signs are absent, further investigation with electro-physiology, quantitative sensory testing, and so on may be required.

5.6 **Mechanisms of neuropathic pain**

Pain is an unpleasant, subjective, sensory, and emotional experience (affective and cognitive components). Psychosocial factors play an important role in its perception and expression. Neuropathic pain, unlike nociceptive pain, is caused by dysfunction of the peripheral or central nervous system, and does not require any receptor stimulation. Small myelinated A-δ and unmyelinated C fibres relay painful symptoms. Unmyelinated C fibres are thought to transmit the slower component of pain, whereas myelinated A-δ fibres relay the faster component.

Table 5.1 shows some of the postulated mechanisms for painful neuropathy, although the complete picture in diabetes is still lacking. There are few clinical studies comparing painful and painless diabetic neuropathy. Clinical and neurophysiological tests are not able to separate painful from painless DPN. Moreover, on the basis of sural nerve morphometry (histology), there are no difference between painful and painless DPN (5). However, a recent in vivo study reported an increase in sural nerve epineurial blood flow in subjects with painful diabetic neuropathy compared to those with painless DPN (6). This suggests that haemodynamic factors may have an important role in the pathogenesis of neuropathic pain and might offer further insight into potential treatments for this distressing condition. Another recent study by Sorensen et al. examined lower limb skin intra-epidermal nerve fibres (IENFs) to evaluate the role of small nerve fibres in the genesis of neuropathic pain (7). They found that more severe loss of IENF is associated with the presence of neuropathic pain in subjects with early neuropathy (7). This finding is supported by the finding of impaired foot skin vasoconstrictor response in patients with painful DPN (8). Another recent study showed increased glycaemic flux in those with painful diabetic neuropathy compared with painless neuropathy (9).

Table 5.1 Mechanisms of neuropathic pain (adapted from ref. 4)	
Peripheral mechanisms	**Central mechanisms**
• Changes in sodium channel distribution and expression	• Central sensitization
• Altered neuropeptide expression	• A fibre sprouting into lamina II of the dorsal horn
• Sympathetic sprouting	• Reduced inhibition of descending pathways
• Peripheral sensitization	
• Altered peripheral blood flow	
• Axonal atrophy, degeneration, or regeneration	
• Damage to small fibres	
• Glycaemic flux	

5.6.1 Central nervous system involvement

Though still known as diabetic 'peripheral' neuropathy, evidence is emerging that DPN may have central manifestations. There is now magnetic resonance imaging (MRI) evidence for the involvement of the spinal cord (10) in DPN and this appears to be early (11). Lesions in the spinal cord may result in pain syndromes similar to those seen after spinal cord injury or demyelination (4). In some patients with painful neuropathy, there may be little in the way of abnormalities on clinical examination or electrophysiological parameters, but there may be evidence of marked abnormalities in somatosensory evoked potentials within the spinal cord (4). Recently, a study using magnetic resonance spectroscopy (MRS) has also demonstrated the presence of thalamic neuronal dysfunction in painless but not painful DPN, suggesting that a functioning thalamus, the gateway to all sensory information, is required in order to perceive pain (4). It is thus increasingly clear that the impact of diabetes on the nervous system is far more generalized than previously thought.

5.6.2 Advances in pain imaging

Recent advances in neuroimaging methods have led to better understanding and refinement of how pain is represented in the cerebral cortex. Early descriptions of pain pathways in humans consisted of relatively simple connections from primary nociceptors to spinal cord and to thalamus, finally terminating in the cerebral cortex. Functional MRI (fMRI) and positron emission tomography studies have subsequently modified this 'hard-wired circuits' view to a more plastic and integrative model, revealing that pain is so much more than sensation.

One of the scientific developments that fuelled the recent advance in our understanding of the function of the human brain has been fMRI. Studies based on fMRI have investigated changes in brain activity in response to various experimental stimuli inducing pain. This has led to the characterization of a network of brain areas that consistently activate in response to pain, forming a 'pain matrix' (12). These cortical and sub-cortical brain networks (regions) comprise the primary and secondary somatosensory cortices, the insular cortex, the anterior cingulate cortex, the thalamus, and the prefrontal cortex. These regions are primarily responsible for discriminating location and intensity of painful stimuli together with affective pain processing. Disruption of the cortical and sub-cortical brain regions that form the pain matrix, and the pathways between them, are thought to have implications for the pathogenesis and persistence of neuropathic pain. These studies, however, have been performed mainly in healthy volunteers following acute pain stimulation, and changes in the brain associated with chronic pain in the context of diabetes need to be investigated.

5.7 Management of painful DPN

The pharmacological management of painful diabetic neuropathy has recently been reviewed by a consensus panel of experts including diabetologists, neurologists, and pain specialists (1). Despite the lack of randomized controlled studies, there is a general consensus that intensive blood glucose control should be the first step in the treatment of any form of diabetic polyneuropathy, including painful DPN. In addition, a major prospective study has implicated traditional markers of large vessel disease including hypertension, obesity, hyperlipidaemia, and smoking in the pathogenesis of DPN (13) and these, therefore need to be effectively managed by life style modifications and drug treatment.

Pharmacological treatment of painful diabetic neuropathy. Box 5.2 shows the range of pharmacological treatments for painful diabetic neuropathy (note some are unlicensed indications).

Only two (duloxetine and pregabalin) are formally approved for the treatment of painful DPN by the FDA. It has to be recognized that treatment usually does not completely abolish the pain. Pain reduction of over 50% is considered clinically significant.

Box 5.2 Pharmacological treatment of painful DPN

- Tight glucose control (HbA1c 6%–7%)
- Life style modification with diet and exercise
- Tricyclic antidepressants (TCAs)
  - Amitriptyline 25–150 mg/day;
  - Imipramine 25–150 mg/day
- Serotonin noradrenaline reuptake inhibitors (SNRIs)
Duloxetine 60–120 mg/day
Venlafaxine 150–225 mg/day
- Anticonvulsants
  - Gabapentin 900–3600 mg/day
  - Pregabalin 300–600 mg/day
  - Carbamazepine up to 800 mg/day
- Opiates
  - Tramadol 200–400 mg/day
  - Oxycodone 20–80 mg/day
  - Morphine sulphate M/r 10–80 mg/day
- IV lidocaine
  - 5 mg/kg given IV over 30 mins with electrocardiogram (ECG) monitoring
- Capsaicin cream
  - (0.075% applied sparingly 3–4 times per day)

5.7.1 **Tricyclic antidepressants**

TCAs relieve pain by inhibiting the re-uptake of 5-HT, noradrenaline, and also by blocking sodium and calcium channels. Several randomized controlled trials have demonstrat0065d the efficacy of TCAs in painful DPN (1). However, TCAs also have many side effects including antimuscarinic effects such as dry mouth, sweating, sedation, and dizziness. Treatment is ideally started with a small dose (10 to 25 mg) of either amitriptyline or imipramine at night, as there is nocturnal exacerbation of painful symptoms and will assist with sleep. The dose can then be gradually titrated depending on adverse events and efficacy. Care should be taken not to exacerbate symptoms of postural hypotension such as dizziness in those with autonomic neuropathy. In addition, a recent data from a retrospective study including 58,956 person years follow-up on TCA therapy indicate an increased risk of sudden cardiac death associated with TCA doses in excess of 100 mg/day (1). Thus, there is a good rationale for not prescribing TCAs to diabetic patients with cardiovascular disease.

5.7.2 **Serotonin noradrenaline reuptake inhibitors**

SNRIs such as duloxetine relieve pain by increasing synaptic availability of 5-HT and noradrenaline in the descending pathways that are inhibitory to pain impulses. The efficacy of duloxetine in painful DPN has been investigated in three identical trials (1; 14) and pooled data from these shows that the 60 and 120 mg/day doses are effective in relieving painful symptoms, starting within a week (Figure 5.1). Efficacy was maintained throughout the treatment period of 12 weeks, and 45%–55% of patients achieved ≥50% pain reduction (1).

The number needed to treat (NNT) to achieve at least 50% pain reduction (clinically meaningful pain reduction) was 4.9 for 120 mg/day, and 5.2 for 60 mg/day (1). A particular advantage of duloxetine was that there was no weight gain during prolonged treatment of up to a year.

In a 6-week trial comparing venlafaxine 75 mg/day and 150 to 225 mg/day with placebo, in 244 diabetic patients with painful DPN, there was significant pain relief in the higher dose group but not in the lower dose (75 mg/day) (1). Side effects included somnolence, nausea, hypertension, and rather worryingly seven patients treated with venlafaxine developed clinically significant ECG changes (1). This is a major concern as many diabetic patients have co-existent cardiac disease. Venlafaxine is currently not licensed for use in painful DPN.

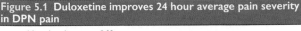

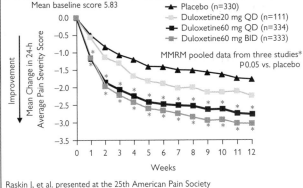

Figure 5.1 Duloxetine improves 24 hour average pain severity in DPN pain

Mean baseline score 5.83

- Placebo (n=330)
- Duloxetine 20 mg QD (n=111)
- Duloxetine 60 mg QD (n=334)
- Duloxetine 60 mg BID (n=333)

MMRM pooled data from three studies*
P 0.05 vs. placebo

Raskin J, et al. presented at the 25th American Pain Society (APS) Annual Scientific Meeting; San Antonio, TX; May 3—6, 2006.

5.7.3 Anticonvulsants

Anticonvulsants inhibit pain by either blocking sodium channels or binding to calcium ion channels. Gabapentin and pregabalin bind to the α-2-δ subunit of the calcium channel reducing calcium flux, and thus resulting in reduced neurotransmitter release in the hyperexcited neurone.

The efficacy of gabapentin in painful DPN comes from one study comparing gabapentin, titrated from 900 to 3600 mg/day over 4 weeks followed with another 4 weeks at the maximum dose, with placebo (1). The 59.5% in the treatment arm, 67% of whom received the highest dose of gabapentin, achieved ≥50% reduction in pain compared with 32.9% with placebo.

Evidence for the efficacy of pregabalin in painful DPN is even better as there have been several clinical trials in painful DPN that demonstrated its efficacy compared to placebo (1). One study looked at a combined analysis of six controlled trials of 5 to 12 weeks duration, and found 39% and 46% of patients with painful DPN treated with pregabalin 300 and 600 mg/day, respectively, achieved at least 50% pain relief (1). Data from seven clinical trials involving pregabalin showed an NNT of 4.04 for 600 mg/day and 5.99 for 300 mg/day (15).

Figure 5.2 Pregbalin: proportion of patients meeting ≥50% and ≥30% improvement

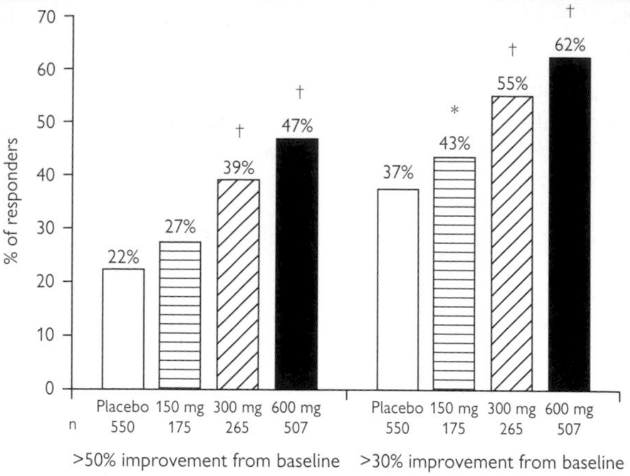

Adapted from Freeman, et al. Diabetes Care 2008; **31**: 1448–54.

5.7.4 **Opioid agonists**

Opioid agonists modulate pain by acting various levels including at the peripheral nociceptor, presynaptic receptor, enkephalin interneurons, post-synaptic receptors, and on the descending systems.

The opiate derivative tramadol has been found effective in relieving neuropathic pain (1). Another opioid, oxycodone slow release has also been shown effective in the management of neuropathic pain (1).

Traditionally clinicians have been rather conservative in the use of opioid agonists, prescribing them as an add-on to other therapy, although clinical evidence to support this approach is somewhat limited. In one cross-over study, low-dose combination therapy with gabapentin and Morphine was significantly more effective than either monotherapy at a higher dose (16). However, combination treatment was associated with a higher frequency of adverse effects than monotherapy (16). Prolonged-release oxycodone was also found to enhance the effects of existing gabapentin therapy in patients with painful DPN (17).

5.7.5 **Topical capsaicin**

Topical capsaicin works by depleting substance 'P' from nerve terminals, and there may be worsening of neuropathic symptoms for the first 2 to 4 weeks of application. Topical capsaicin (0.075%) applied sparingly 3 to 4 times per day to the affected area has also been found to relieve neuropathic pain.

5.7.6 Lacosamide

Lacosamide is promising anticonvulsant for the treatment of painful DPN. In a phase-2 study, lacosamide was found to be beneficial in relieving painful DPN but phase 3 studies are now required.

5.7.7 α-Lipoic acid

Infusion of the antioxidant α-lipoic acid at a dose of 600 mg intravenously per day over a 3-week period has been found to be useful in reducing neuropathic pain (1). A meta-analysis including 1258 patients from four prospective trials showed that treatment with α-lipoic acid (600 mg/day) for 3 weeks was associated with significant and clinically meaningful improvement in positive neuropathic symptoms (pain, burning, paraesthesia, and numbness), as well as neuropathic deficits (1). Oral treatment with α-lipoic acid for 5 weeks improved neuropathic symptoms and deficits in patients with DPN (18). An oral dose of 600 mg once daily appears to provide the optimum risk-to-benefit ratio (18), but a confirmatory larger trial may be required.

5.8 Comparison of the efficacy and safety

A way of comparing across the range of the various treatments is by estimation of the NNT and number needed to harm (NNH) (1). The NNT is defined as the number of patients needed to treat with a certain drug to obtain one patient with 50% pain relief (1). The NNH is defined as the number of patients needs to be treated for one patient to drop out of a study as a result of adverse effects (1). Though this is a useful approach, it has drawbacks as many of the trials have different designs, end points, and so on, and one is not comparing like with like.

Figure 5.3 shows the NNTs for the various drugs in painful neuropathy including painful DPN. The size of circles corresponds to the total number of patients used in trials. TCAs have the lowest NNTs (1). However, some of the clinical trials were cross over, and that is likely to lower the NNT. TCAs also have increased risk of adverse side effects, including sedation, dry mouth, sweating, dizziness, as well as contraindications, for use in heart disease, epilepsy, and glaucoma (1). The largest number of patients in trials involved pregabalin, duloxetine, and gabapentin, and these compounds appear to have similar intermediate efficacy (Figure 5.3). Nausea is more common for duloxetine (1) whilst dizziness and somnolence are more common for pregabalin and gabapentin (1).

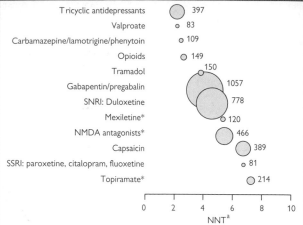

Figure 5.3 Proposed treatment algorithm for painful diabetic neuropathy. Adapted from ref. (1)

Tricyclic antidepressants — 397
Valproate — 83
Carbamazepine/lamotrigine/phenytoin — 109
Opioids — 149
Tramadol — 150
Gabapentin/pregabalin — 1057
SNRI: Duloxetine — 778
Mexiletine* — 120
NMDA antagonists* — 466
Capsaicin — 389
SSRI: paroxetine, citalopram, fluoxetine — 81
Topiramate* — 214

NNT^a

^{a} NNT was defined as the number of patients needed to treat (NNT) to obtain one patient with 50% pain relief

* At least half of the conducted trials showed no significant effect and this drug has been discontinued by manufacturers in the UK.

Key: SNRI = selective serotonin and noradrenaline re-uptake inhibitor;
NMDA = N-methyl-D-aspartate; SSRI = selective serotonin re-uptake inhibitor
Note : Some of these are unlincensed uses.

5.9 Treatment algorithm

A recent consensus meeting carefully evaluated the trial evidence for the various pharmacological treatments for painful DPN and suggested a treatment algorithm (1) (Figure 5.3). The panel compared of the relative efficacy and safety of treatments for painful DPN, based on the available NNT for neuropathic pain (including painful DPN) and NNH data, and recommended that a TCA, SNRI, or an α-2-δ agonist should be considered for first-line treatment of painful DPN (Figure 5.3). On the basis of trial data, duloxetine, the preferred SNRI, and pregabalin would be the preferred α-2-δ agonist. Initial selection of appropriate treatment may depend on assessment of comorbidities and contraindications as well as cost. In diabetic patients with a history of heart disease, in elderly patients on other concomitant medications such as diuretics and antihypertensives, in patients with co-morbid orthostatic hypotension, and so on, TCAs have relative contraindication. In those with liver disease duloxetine should not be prescribed, and in those with oedema pregabalin or gabapentin should be avoided. A simple questionnaire (verbal descriptor scale, e.g. 'none, mild, moderate, and severe') or preferably a visual analogue scale may assist in the monitoring treatment response. If pain is inadequately controlled, depending on contraindications, a different first-line agent may be considered as shown in Figure 5.3.

Combination of first-line therapies may be considered if there is pain, despite a change in first-line monotherapy (Figure 5.3). If pain is inadequately controlled, opioids such as tramadol and oxycodone may be added in a combination treatment. Opiates should be avoided in those with a history of substance misuse.

5.10 **Non-pharmacological treatments**

Lack of response and unwanted side effects of conventional drug treatments force many sufferers to try alternative therapies such as acupuncture (4), near-infrared phototherapy (4), low-intensity laser therapy (4), magnetic field therapies (4), and transcutaneous electrical stimulation (TENS) (4), frequency-modulated electromagnetic neural stimulation (FREMS) therapy (4), high-frequency external muscle stimulation (4) and as a last resort, implantation of electrical spinal cord stimulator (19).

5.10.1 **Electrical spinal cord stimulation**

Neuropathic pain can sometimes be extremely severe, interfering significantly with patients' sleep and daily activities. Unfortunately, some patients are not helped by conventional pharmacological treatment. Such patients pose a major challenge for they are severely distressed and sometimes wheelchair bound. The last option for such patients is electrical spinal cord stimulation which has been found to relieve both background and peak neuropathic pain (19) in DPN. This form of treatment is particularly advantageous, as the patient may not require any other pain-relieving medications, with all their side effects. Clearly as the procedure is invasive, it is reserved as a last option and is available in specialist centres. A recent follow-up of patients fitted with electrical spinal cord stimulators found that stimulators continued to be effective 10 years after implantation.

49

5.11 **Conclusions**

1. Pain is the most distressing symptom of DPN and the main reason seeking medical attention.
2. Painful DPN is a significant clinical problem affecting 10%–20% of all diabetic patients. Despite this in one study 12.5% had never reported their symptoms to their physician and 39.3% had never received any treatment for their pain (20). Thus painful DPN continues to be under-diagnosed and under-treated and this unsatisfactory scenario must change.

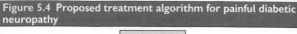

Figure 5.4 Proposed treatment algorithm for painful diabetic neuropathy

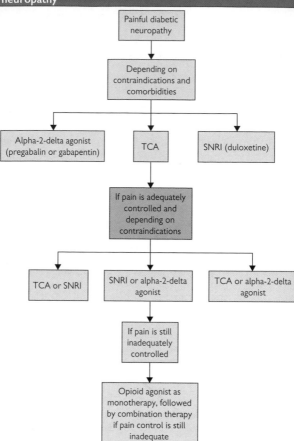

Key: TCA = tricyclic antidepressant; SNRI = selective serotonin noradrenaline re-uptake inhibitor

3. The minimum requirements for diagnosis of painful DPN are assessment of symptoms and neurological examination, with shoes and sock removed. Bilateral sensory impairment is almost always present.

4. Painful diabetic neuropathy is characterized by burning, shooting, or stabbing pain in the extremities. Pain may be spontaneous or evoked.

5. Optimization of cardiovascular risk factors and improved glycaemic control are important.

6. First-line therapies for painful DPN are a TCA, SNRI (such as duloxetine), or anticonvulsants (such as pregabalin or gabapentin), taking into account patients' co-morbidities and cost.

7. Combination therapy may be useful but further research is required.

8. Studies are required on direct head-to-head comparative trials and long-term efficacy of drugs, as most trials have lasted less than 16 weeks.

9. There is also a need for further controlled trials to investigate non-pharmacological treatments.

10. For intractable painful neuropathy that does not respond to any pharmacological and simple non-pharmacological treatments, consider implantable electrical spinal cord stimulator.

References

1. Jensen TS, Backonja MM, Hernandez Jimenez S, Tesfaye S, Valensi P, Ziegler D. New perspectives on the management of diabetic peripheral neuropathic pain. *Diab Vasc Dis Res* 2006; **3**: 108–19.

2. Quattrini C, Tesfaye S. Understanding the impact of painful diabetic neuropathy. *Diabetes Metab Res Rev* 2003; **19**. S2–8.

3. Tesfaye S, Malik R, Harris N et al. Arterio-venous shunting and proliferating new vessels in acute painful neuropathy of rapid glycaemic control (insulin neuritis). *Diabetologia* 1996; **39**: 329–35.

4. Tesfaye S, Kempler P. Painful diabetic neuropathy. *Diabetologia* 2005; **48**: 805–7.

5. Britland ST, Young RJ, Sharma AK et al. Acute remitting painful diabetic polyneuropathy: a comparison of peripheral nerve fibre pathology. *Pain* 1992; **48**: 361–70.

6. Eaton SE, Harris ND, Ibrahim S et al. Increased sural nerve epineurial blood flow in human subjects with painful diabetic neuropathy. *Diabetologia* 2003; **46**: 934–9.

7. Sorensen L, Molyneaux L, Yue DK. The relationship among pain, sensory loss, and small nerve fibers in diabetes. *Diabetes Care* 2006; **29**: 883–7.

8. Quattrini C, Harris ND, Malik RA, Tesfaye S. Impaired skin microvascular reactivity in painful diabetic neuropathy. *Diabetes Care* 2007; **30**: 655–9.

9. Oyibo SO, Prasad YD, Jackson NJ, Jude EB, Boulton AJ. The relationship between blood glucose excursions and painful diabetic peripheral neuropathy: a pilot study. *Diabet Med* 2002; **19**(10): 870–3.

10. Eaton S, Harris ND, Rajbhandari SM et al. Spinal cord involvement in diabetic peripheral neuropathy. *Lancet* 2001; **358**: 35–6.

11. Selvarajah D, Wilkinson ID, Emery CJ et al. Early involvement of the spinal cord in diabetic peripheral neuropathy. *Diabetes Care* 2006; **29**: 2664–9.

12. Melzack R. From the gate to the neuromatrix. *Pain* 1999; (Suppl 6): S121–6.

13. Tesfaye S, Chaturvedi N, Eaton SEM, Witte D, Ward JD, Fuller J. Vascular risk factors and diabetic neuropathy. *N Engl J Med* 2005; **352**: 341–50.

14. Goldstein DJ, Lu Y, Detke MJ et al. Duloxetine vs. placebo in patients with painful diabetic neuropathy. *Pain* 2005; **116**: 109–18.

15. Freeman R, Durso-Decruz E, Emir B. Efficacy, safety and tolerability of pregabalin treatment of painful diabetic peripheral neuropathy: findings from 7 randomized, controlled trials across a range of doses. *Diabetes Care* 2008; **31**: 1448–54.

16. Gilron I, Bailey JM, Tu D et al. Morphine, gabapentin, or their combination for neuropathic pain. *N Engl J Med* 2005; **352**: 1324–34.

17. Hanna M, O'Brien C, Wilson MC. Prolonged-release oxycodone enhances the effects of existing gabapentin therapy in painful diabetic neuropathy patients. *Eur J Pain* 2008; **12**(6):804–13.

18 Ziegler D, Ametov A, Barinov A et al. Oral treatment with α-lipoic acid improves symptomatic diabetic polyneuropathy. The SYDNEY 2 trial. *Diabetes Care* 2006; **29**: 2365–70.

19. Tesfaye S, Watt J, Benbow SJ, Pang KA, Miles J, MacFarlane IA. Electrical spinal cord stimulation for painful diabetic peripheral neuropathy. *Lancet* 1996; **348**: 1696–170.

20. Daousi C, MacFarlane IA, Woodward A et al. Chronic painful peripheral neuropathy in an urban community: a controlled comparison of people with and without diabetes. *Diabet Med* 2004; **21**: 976–82.

Chapter 6

Treatment of autonomic dysfunction in peripheral neuropathies

Roy Freeman

Key points

- Autonomic dysfunction causes considerable morbidity and may increase mortality in diabetes.
- Manifestations may affect cardiovascular, urogenital, gastrointestinal, pupillomotor, thermoregulatory, and sudomotor function.
- Some patients will be improved by counselling and non-pharmacological interventions.
- More severely afflicted patients require pharmacological interventions.

6.1 Introduction

The autonomic manifestations of diabetes are responsible for the most troublesome and disabling features of diabetic peripheral neuropathy and result in a significant proportion of the mortality and morbidity associated with the disease. With the help of non-pharmacological and pharmacological interventions, most patients' quality of life can be improved substantially. Some patients will be improved by counselling and non-pharmacological interventions, while others require pharmacological interventions.

6.2 Treatment of orthostatic hypotension

6.2.1 Physiology and pathophysiology

Orthostatic hypotension is the most incapacitating symptom of autonomic dysfunction. A baroreflex-mediated reflex occurs in response to standing which increases peripheral resistance, venous return to the heart and cardiac output, and thus limits the fall in blood pressure.

If this response fails, orthostatic hypotension and cerebral hypoperfusion occur (Figure 6.1).

6.2.2 **Treatment**

6.2.2.1 *Non-pharmacological measures*

- Patient education is the cornerstone of the management of orthostatic hypotension. Patients with orthostatic hypotension should move from a supine to standing position in gradual stages. A number of physical manoeuvres that can help maintain blood pressure during daily activities such as leg crossing, stooping, and squatting.

- The excessive natriuresis and reduction in central blood volume can be attenuated or minimized by increasing sodium intake with high sodium containing foods or salt tablets. Patients should have a daily dietary intake of up to 10 g (185 mmol) of sodium chloride per day and a fluid intake of 2 to 2.5 L/day. Raising the head of the bed 10° to 20° activates the renin–angiotensin–aldosterone system and decreases the nocturnal diuresis.

- Ingestion of ~500 mL of tap water elicits a marked pressor response and improvement in symptoms in patients with autonomic failure. The pressor response, a systolic blood pressure increase of over 30 mmHg in some patients, is evident within 5 min after water ingestion.

- The use of custom-fitted elastic stockings permits the application of a graded pressure to the lower extremity and abdomen. It is essential that such stockings extend to the waist as most peripheral pooling occurs in the splanchnic circulation.

- Removal of potential reversible causes of orthostatic hypotension is an important management step. Medications such as diuretics, antihypertensive agents, antianginal agents, alpha-adrenoreceptor antagonists to treat benign prostatic hyperplasia, and antidepressants are the most common offending agents.

6.2.2.2 *Pharmacological measures*

Numerous agents from diverse pharmacological groups have been implemented in the treatment of orthostatic hypotension (See Box 6.1). The therapeutic goal is merely to ameliorate all symptoms while avoiding side effects. There is rarely the need to restore normotension.

6.2.2.2.1 *Agents to increase central blood volume*

9-α-Fluorohydrocortisone

9-α-Fluorohydrocortisone (fludrocortisone acetate), a synthetic mineralocorticoid, can be used to supplement the increase in dietary fluids and salt. Fludrocortisone increases the blood volume and may enhance the sensitivity of blood vessels to circulating catecholamines.

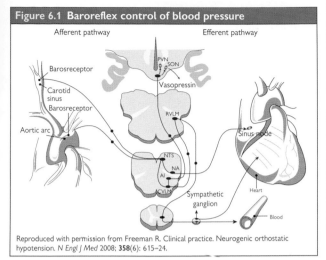

Figure 6.1 Baroreflex control of blood pressure

Afferent pathway   Efferent pathway

Baroreceptor

Carotid sinus

Baroreceptor

Aortic arc

PVN

SON

Vasopressin

RVLM

NTS

NA

AI

CVLM

Sympathetic ganglion

Sinus node

Heart

Blood

Reproduced with permission from Freeman R. Clinical practice. Neurogenic orthostatic hypotension. *N Engl J Med* 2008; **358**(6): 615–24.

Treatment is initiated with a 0.1 mg tablet daily. Treatment may be limited by supine hypertension, ankle oedema, hypokalaemia, and rarely congestive heart failure. Potassium supplementation is usually required, particularly when higher doses are used.

Vasopressin analogues

The synthetic vasopressin analogue desmopressin acetate may also be used to enhance fluid retention in patients with orthostatic hypotension. Desmopressin, which can be taken as a nasal spray (10 to 40 mcg) or orally (100 to 800 mcg), may prevent the nocturia, and reduces the morning postural fall in blood pressure in patients with autonomic failure. Fluid and electrolyte status should be carefully monitored during therapy to avoid hyponatraemia.

6.2.2.2.2 Sympathomimetic agents

A direct or indirect sympathomimetic agent may be used in conjunction with central blood volume supplementation so that the patient should remain symptomatic.

The peripheral selective α-agonist, midodrine, is the most widely prescribed agent for the treatment of orthostatic hypotension in the USA but is not generally available in the UK. The pressor effect of midodrine is due to both arterial and venous constriction. Dose should be titrated from 2.5 to 10 mg three or four times a day. Potential side effects of this agent include pilomotor reactions, pruritus, supine hypertension, gastrointestinal complaints, and urinary retention. This agent does not cross the blood brain barrier and central nervous system side effects occur infrequently.

55

Box 6.1 Agents for the treatment of orthostatic hypotension

- Mineralocorticoids
  - 9-α-Fludrocortisone
- Sympathomimetic agents
  - Midodrine
  - Ephedrine
  - Pseudoephedrine
  - Phenylephrine
  - Methylphenidate
  - Dextroamphetamine
  - Tyramine (with monoamine oxidase inhibition)
  - Clonidine
  - Yohimbine
  - DL- and L-dihydroxyphenylserine (DL-DOPS)
- Non-specific pressor agents
  - Ergot derivatives
  - Caffeine
  - Somatostatin analogues
- β-Adrenergic blocking agents
  - Propranolol
  - Pindolol
  - Xamoterol
  - Prenalterol
- Dopamine blocking agents
  - Metoclopramide
  - Domperidone
- V1 and V2 receptor agonists
  - Desmopressin acetate
  - Lysine–vasopressin
- Erythropoietin

Note: Some of these agents are not licensed and may be unavailable in the UK.

Ephedrine (25 to 50 mg three times a day) and pseudoephedrine (30 to 60 mg three times a day) are the most frequently prescribed indirectly acting agents. Adverse events associated with these agents include supine hypertension, tachycardia, central sympathomimetic side effects (e.g. anxiety, tremulousness) and rarely intracerebral haemorrhage, vasculitis, arrhythmias, and cardiovascular events. Abuse potential exists for these agents.

Erythropoietin

Erythropoietin increases standing blood pressure and improves orthostatic tolerance in patients with orthostatic hypotension. This agent corrects the normochromic normocytic anaemia that frequently accompanies autonomic failure. Recombinant human erythropoietin is administered subcutaneously or intravenously at doses between 25 and 75 U/kg three times a week until a haematocrit that approaches normal is attained. Adverse events include polycythaemia and cardiovascular events. The long-term risks in this patient population are not known.

6.2.2.2.3 Other agents

A list of some other agents that have been used in the treatment of orthostatic hypotension is present in Box 6.1. Evidence in support of these agents is limited.

6.3 Treatment of bowel dysfunction

6.3.1 Physiology and pathophysiology

The autonomic control of the gastrointestinal tract is mediated by the extrinsic parasympathetic and sympathetic nervous systems and the intrinsic enteric nervous system. The degeneration of both extrinsic and intrinsic autonomic neurons in patients with autonomic neuropathy results in symptoms of gastrointestinal dysfunction that involve both the upper and the lower gastrointestinal tract. The symptoms of upper gastrointestinal autonomic dysfunction are exemplified by the features of gastroparesis diabeticorum: abdominal bloating, postprandial fullness, early satiety, nausea, and vomiting occur commonly in diabetic patients. Other upper gastrointestinal features include gastrocsophageal reflux disorder and dysphagia while constipation, abdominal fullness, diarrhoea, and faecal incontinence are the hallmarks of lower gastrointestinal tract dysfunction (4–6).

6.3.2 Diabetic gastroparesis

The true prevalence of diabetic gastroparesis is not known; up to 40% of diabetic patients may develop gastroparesis. The diagnosis is made when the characteristic symptom complex is accompanied by delayed gastric emptying in the absence of a mechanical obstructive lesion.

6.3.2.1 Treatment of diabetic gastroparesis

Glucose control should be optimized in patients with gastroparesis as hyperglycaemia may delay gastric emptying. Some medications may impair gastric emptying and should be discontinued if possible. These include antihypertensives such as calcium-channel blockers; oral anti-hyperglycaemic agents such as the incretin, exenatide; and antimuscarinic agents such as antispasmodic agents and antidepressants. Frequent small meals and the consumption of homogenized food may be sufficient to control symptoms in some patients. More severely afflicted patients may require pharmacotherapy. The prokinetic medications are the primary pharmacological agents used to treat this disorder (Box 6.2).

Box 6.2 Pharmacotherapy of gastroparesis

- Prokinetic agents
  - Metoclopramide
  - Domperidone
  - Erythromycin
  - Cholinomimetics
  —Bethanechol
  —Acetylcholinesterase inhibitors
  - Cisapride (discontinued)
- Antiemetic agents
  - Histamine (H1) receptor antagonists
  - Serotonin (5HT3) receptor antagonists
  - Dopamine (D2) receptor antagonists
- Decompression, surgery, and experimental procedures
  - Gastrostomy or jejunostomy
  - Surgery
  - Botulinum toxin type A
  - Gastric pacing

Prokinetic agents

The benzamide, metoclopramide (10 mg tid orally, 30 min before meals and at bedtime), accelerates gastric emptying, and also has a central antiemetic action. The prokinetic effects are due to augmented release of acetylcholine from enteric cholinergic neurons (due to activation of 5HT4 receptors) and dopamine (D2) receptor antagonism. The central antiemetic effects of metoclopramide are mediated by dopamine (D2) receptor and serotonin (5HT3) receptor antagonism in the area postrema of the peri-aqueductal grey. Patients maintained in the long term on metoclopramide may be at risk for the development of tardive dyskinesia and other dopamine-antagonist-related side effects.

Erythromycin, administered both orally (250 mg tid) and intravenously (3 mg/kg every 8 h), improves gastric emptying and gastroparetic symptoms. This agent and related macrolide compounds exhibit strong *in vitro* affinity for motilin receptors, and have agonist properties that mimic the prokinetic action of exogenous motilin, a gastrointestinal polypeptide. However, erythromycin is currently an unlicensed and unproven treatment, lacking strong trial evidence.

Domperidone is a D_2 receptor antagonist that does not cross the blood brain barrier. While this drug has no central anti-dopaminergic effects, some central antiemetic effects may be due to activity in the area postrema. This agent is not available in the USA. Typical doses are 10 to 20 mg tid.

Muscarinic cholinergic agonists for example bethanechol (10 to 20 mg tid) and acetylcholinesterase inhibitors such as pyridostigmine (30 mg qid) may be helpful in some patients.

Cisapride is a cholinomimetic agent which increases motility in oesophagus, stomach, and bowel by enhancing release of acetylcholine from neurons of the myenteric plexus. These effects are mediated by $5HT_4$ receptor agonism. Due to an increased incidence of ventricular arrhythmias including torsade de pointes, this agent is no longer available for general use. A limited access compassionate use programme for use of this agent is available for patients who are refractory to all medications.

Antiemetic agents

Antiemetic agents may supplement pharmacotherapy with prokinetic agents. Commonly used agents include the histamine (H1) receptor antagonists [e.g. dimenhydrinate (50 mg tid)], the serotonin (5HT3) receptor antagonists [e.g. odansetron (4 to 8 mg tid)], and the dopamine (D2) receptor antagonists [e.g. prochlorperazine (5 to 10 mg tid)].

6.3.2.2 *Decompression, surgery, and experimental procedures*

Percutaneous or laparoscopic gastrostomy or jejunostomy may be required in patients' refractory to pharmacological intervention. Surgery is rarely required.

Botulinum toxin type A has been used to treat refractory gastroparesis. The dose of botulinum has ranged from 80 to 200 units, injected directly into the pylorus. Several small case studies and open-label trials have suggested efficacy in patients' refractory to standard management, although this has not been confirmed in controlled studies.

Gastric pacing may be considered as a last resort. Gastric electrical stimulation may be considered in patients who are refractory to all medical intervention. This service is available in some specialist centres in Europe and the USA (Box 6.3).

Box 6.3 Gastric electrical stimulation

- May significantly improve nausea and vomiting, quality of life, and glycaemic control but does not improve gastric emptying
- There is a post-operative infection rate of around 10% and there may be some evidence for cost effectiveness
- Almost all evidence is from uncontrolled studies and RCTs are required to confirm these findings

---

6.3.3 **Bowel hypomotility**

Constipation is the most frequently reported gastrointestinal auto-nomic symptom and is found in up to 60% of diabetics (9). The pathophysiology of diabetic constipation is poorly understood but may reflect intestinal denervation and loss of the post-prandial gastro-colic reflex. Several studies have documented prolonged colonic transit times in diabetic patients with constipation.

6.3.4 **Treatment of bowel hypomotility**

An increase in dietary fibre (up to 25 g/day) with water (300 mL four times per day) and exercise is the first line of therapy for most patients. The use of psyllium (up to 30 g/day), not normally avail-able in UK, or methylcellulose (up to 6 g/day) with a concomitant increase in fluid intake will further increase stool bulk. These agents and fibre should be increased gradually and concomitantly with an increase in fluid ingestion.

Stool softeners (e.g. docusate sodium 100 to 500 mg/day) or lubri-cants (e.g. mineral oil) together with an osmotic laxative (e.g. magne-sium sulphate, magnesium citrate, polyethylene glycol, and lactulose 15 to 60 mL/day) may be used if the above measures are ineffective, but are to be avoided if possible. Glycerine suppositories or sodium phosphate enemas stimulate evacuation by promoting fluid retention in the rectum (see Box 6.4).

The contact cathartics, such as the diphenylmethane derivatives (phenolphthalein and bisacodyl), the anthraquinones (senna and cascara) should be used sparingly, although the use of these agents often cannot be avoided in patients with constipation due to severe autonomic dysfunction.

Other agents that may be helpful include the synthetic prostaglandin E1 analogue, misoprostol, the neurotrophin, NT_3, and the chloride channel activator, lubiprostone (available in the USA but not in the UK). The $5HT_4$ partial agonist, tegaserod, was removed from the market in 2007 due to cardiovascular adverse effects.

6.3.5 **Diabetic diarrhoea**

Diabetic diarrhoea manifests as a profuse, watery, typically nocturnal diarrhoea which can last for hours or days and frequently alternates with constipation. Abdominal discomfort is commonly associated. The pathogenesis of diabetic diarrhoea includes reduced gastrointes-tinal motility, reduced receptor-mediated fluid absorption, bacterial overgrowth, pancreatic insufficiency, co-existent celiac disease, and abnormalities in bile salt metabolism. Treatment with the oral anti-hyperglycaemic agent, metformin, should also be considered. Faecal incontinence, due to anal sphincter incompetence or reduced rectal sensation, is often exacerbated by diarrhoea.

Box 6.4 Pharmacotherapy of bowel hypomotility used internationally

- Bulk agents
  - Bran
  - Psyllium
  - Methylcellulose
- Laxatives and cathartics:
  - Osmotic laxatives and cathartics
  —Lactulose
  —Sorbitol
  —Magnesium salts
  —Sodium phosphate
  —Polyethylene glycol–saline solutions
  —Glycerine suppositories
  - Contact cathartics
  —Diphenylmethane derivatives
    —Phenolphthalein
    —Bisacodyl tablets or suppositories
  —Anthraquinone derivatives
    —Senna
    —Cascara
  - Ricinoleic acid (Castor oil)
- Stool softeners and lubricants:
  - Mineral oil
  - Docusates
- Prokinetic agents
  - Metoclopramide
  - Cisapride
  - Domperidone
  - Erythromycin
  - Cholinomimetics
  —Bethanechol
  —Acetyl cholinesterase inhibitors
  - Opioid antagonists
  - Misoprostol
  - Lubiprostone

61

6.3.5.1 *Treatment of diabetic diarrhoea*

Treatment of diabetic diarrhoea should be directed at the underlying cause. If bacterial overgrowth is suspected, a trial of antibiotic therapy (e.g. tetracyclines, metronidazole, or a cephalosporin) should be conducted especially when steatorrhoea is present. Bile acid malabsorption may be treated with colestyramine.

The anti-diarrhoeal synthetic opioids [loperamide (2 to 4 mg four times daily), co-phenotrope (diphenoxylate and atropine) (2 tablets four times daily), and codeine (30 mg four times daily)] are the most widely used agents. These agents decrease peristalsis and increase rectal sphincter tone.

There is empirical evidence suggesting that the alpha-2-adrenergic receptor agonist, clonidine, may be of benefit in the treatment of diarrhoea in doses of up to 1.2 mg/day. The proposed mechanism to explain the efficacy of this agent is dysregulation of alpha-2-adrenoreceptor-mediated intestinal ion transport in diabetic diarrhoea.

The long-acting somatostatin analogue, octreotide (50 to 75 mcg bid or tid), may be of benefit in refractory patients. This agent suppresses gastrointestinal motility and inhibits the release of peptides such as motilin, serotonin, and gastrin. Concerning adverse events associated with this agent include recurrent hypoglycaemia due to impaired counter-regulation and abdominal cramps.

In addition, treatment with prokinetic agents (see earlier) may paradoxically improve diarrhoea in some patients.

In the individual case, empiric management with antibiotics, synthetic opioids, prokinetic agents, psyllium, antimuscarinics, somatostatin, and others agents is often required.

6.4 **Treatment of bladder hypomotility**

6.4.1 **Physiology and pathophysiology**

Symptoms of bladder dysfunction have been observed in 37%–50% of diabetic patients and there is physiologic evidence of bladder dysfunction in 43%–87% of insulin-dependent diabetic patients. Bladder symptoms associated with autonomic neuropathy include hesitancy, poor stream, increased intervals between micturition, prolonged bladder emptying, and a sense of inadequate bladder emptying. These symptoms may be followed by urinary retention and overflow incontinence.

The bladder wall is comprised of three layers of interdigitating smooth muscle and serves as a receptacle for the storage and appropriate evacuation of urine. This smooth muscle—the detrusor muscle—forms the internal sphincter at the junction of the bladder neck and urethra while the external sphincter is formed from the striated muscle of the urogenital diaphragm and is a true anatomical sphincter. The bladder has parasympathetic, sympathetic, and somatic innervation.

6.4.2 **Therapy of bladder hypomotility**

Initial therapy should emphasize timed voiding schedules with bladder contractions enhanced by a Valsalva manoeuvre and Credé manoeuvre. Clean intermittent self-catheterization, however, is the primary therapy for impaired or absent detrusor muscle activity. The interval between catheterizations should be designed to maintain a residual volume of less than 100 mL and avoid incontinence. The majority of patients performing self-catheterization will develop bacteriuria; however, antibiotic therapy is only necessary if symptomatic urinary tract infections occur. Long-term catheterization is rarely necessary. Adverse effects of long-term catheterization include infections, meatal erosions in males, and vaginal fistulas in females.

Pharmacotherapy has a very limited role in the treatment of detrusor areflexia. Stimulation of muscarinic, post-ganglionic receptors results in enhanced bladder contractility. Bethanechol chloride is a parasympathomimetic drug with relatively selective action at the urinary bladder. This agent may be effective in chronic states of detrusor atony or hypotonicity. Typical oral doses range from 25 to 100 mg four times daily (this is above normal maximum dose). There is insufficient evidence to warrant routine use of this agent in the treatment of detrusor hypomotility.

References

1. Camilleri M. Clinical practice. Diabetic gastroparesis. *N Engl J Med* 2007; **356**(8): 820–9.

2. Chandrasekharan B, Srinivasan S. Diabetes and the enteric nervous system. *Neurogastroenterol Motil* 2007; **19**(12): 951–60.

3. Fedele D. Therapy Insight: sexual and bladder dysfunction associated with diabetes mellitus. *Nat Clin Pract Urol* 2005; **2**(6): 282–90.

4. Feldman M, Schiller LR. Disorders of gastrointestinal motility associated with diabetes mellitus. *Ann Intern Med* 1983; **98**: 378–84.

5. Fowler CJ, Griffiths D, de Groat WC. The neural control of micturition. *Nat Rev Neurosci* 2008; **9**(6): 453–66.

6. Fowler CJ. Neurological disorders of micturition and their treatment. *Brain* 1999; **122**(Pt 7): 1213–31.

7. Freeman R. Current pharmacologic treatment for orthostatic hypotension. *Clin Auton Res* 2008; **18**(Suppl 1):14–8.

8. Lembo A, Camilleri M. Chronic constipation. *N Engl J Med* 2003; **349**(14): 1360–8.

9. Low PA, Singer W. Management of neurogenic orthostatic hypotension: an update. *Lancet Neurol* 2008; **7**(5): 451–8.

10. Maleki D, Locke GR, III, Camilleri M *et al.* Gastrointestinal tract symptoms among persons with diabetes mellitus in the community. *Arch Intern Med* 2000; **160**(18): 2808–16.

11. Park MI, Camilleri M. Gastroparesis: clinical update. *Am J Gastroenterol* 2006; **101**(5): 1129–39.

12. Schiller LR. Management of diarrhea in clinical practice: strategies for primary care physicians. *Rev Gastroenterol Disord* 2007; **7** (Suppl 3): S27–38.

13. Sellin JH, Chang EB. Therapy insight: gastrointestinal complications of diabetes—pathophysiology and management. *Nat Clin Pract Gastroenterol Hepatol* 2008; **5**(3): 162–71.

14. Smit AA, Halliwill JR, Low PA, Wieling W. Pathophysiological basis of orthostatic hypotension in autonomic failure. *J Physiol* 1999; **519**(Pt 1): 1–10.

Chapter 7

The management of erectile dysfunction

David E Price

Key points
• Impotence is a distressing problem which affects 30%–40% of diabetic men.
• Tumescence occurs as a result of nitric oxide (NO)-mediated smooth muscle relaxation of the erectile tissue leading to engorgement of the corpus cavernosum.
• Erection is initiated by neuronal NO release and maintained by NO released by the local vascular endothelium.
• Impotence in diabetes occurs as a result of endothelial dysfunction and autonomic neuropathy.
• Phosphodiesterase 5 (PDE5) inhibitors are used for the first-line treatment of impotence in diabetes and are effective in 50% to 60% of diabetic men.

7.1 Introduction

Erectile dysfunction (ED) is a common and distressing problem in diabetic men. Although autonomic neuropathy plays an important role in the pathogenesis of ED in diabetes, it is mainly a manifestation of endothelial and vascular dysfunction. However, most diabetic men with clinically apparent neuropathy will have ED and, as it is easy and rewarding to treat, it is entirely appropriate that a chapter on ED is included in this book.

7.2 Prevalence of ED in diabetes

ED is a common problem in both diabetic and non-diabetic men. A population-based study in Spain reported that diabetes was by far the major risk factor for ED. The prevalence of ED in the overall population was 12.1%. Diabetes increased the risk of ED fourfold, greater than any other risk factor. In a diabetic clinic population, the prevalence of ED is generally reported to be about 35%. All studies have shown that the prevalence of ED increases with age so that after the age of 50 the majority of diabetic men suffer with the problem.

7.3 **Pathophysiology of ED in diabetes**

7.3.1 **Physiology of normal penile erection**

Erections are the result of blood engorging the erectile tissue of the penis which is a vascular sponge lined by endothelial cells and surrounded by smooth muscle cells which is surrounded in turn by the fibrous tunica albuginea. Under conditions of sexual stimulation, there is relaxation of the vascular smooth muscle of the erectile tissue and the inflow arterioles controlled by the autonomic nervous system. The resultant expansion of the erectile tissue causes compression of the outflow venules against the firm tunica albuginea and reduces venous outflow leading to tumescence (Figure 7.1).

Nitric oxide (NO), derived from both parasympathetic fibres and the vascular endothelium, plays a central role in the whole process. A model of our current understanding is shown in Figure 7.2. There is some evidence that neuronally derived NO is important in initiation, whereas NO from the endothelium is responsible for maintenance of erection.

Tumescence results from NO released directly from nerve terminals and from NO released from endothelial cells under autonomic control mediated by acetylcholine and there is evidence that in the diabetic

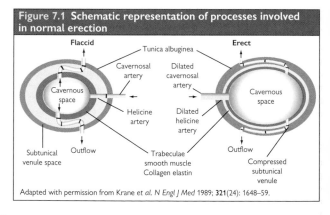

Figure 7.1 Schematic representation of processes involved in normal erection

Flaccid

Tunica albuginea

Cavernosal artery

Cavernous space

Helicine artery

Subtunical venule space

Outflow

Trabeculae smooth muscle
Collagen elastin

Erect

Dilated cavernosal artery

Cavernous space

Dilated helicine artery

Outflow

Compressed subtunical venule

Adapted with permission from Krane et al. N Engl J Med 1989; **321**(24): 1648–59.

subjects both pathways are impaired. In other words, impotence in diabetes is secondary to a failure of NO-mediated smooth muscle relaxation due to both autonomic neuropathy and endothelial dysfunction. Many diabetic men report that in the early stages they do not have a problem initially achieving an erection but that they cannot maintain it. This would suggest that in these individuals failure of endothelium-derived NO occurs before significant autonomic neuropathy.

Many other factors contribute to the development of ED in diabetes including large vessel disease and concomitant medication.

7.4 Clinical features and investigation

ED in diabetic men is usually gradual in onset and progressive in nature but the features are variable. The initial problem is usually the inability to sustain an erection long enough for satisfactory intercourse. Spontaneous recovery of erectile function in diabetes is rare. Few investigations are required in the management of a diabetic man with ED. As it is a manifestation of endothelial dysfunction an assessment of cardiovascular risk should be considered which should include measurement of blood pressure, lipid profile, and urinalysis for microalbuminuria. A serum testosterone that should be considered as borderline hypogonadism is common finding in middle-aged and elderly men, and there is some evidence that correction of low serum testosterone can improve the response rate to ED treatments.

7.5 The management of ED in diabetes

7.5.1 General advice

In most cases, diabetologists and general practitioners can provide the common sense advice required without specialist psychosexual counselling. It is important to establish that the couple have maintained a good relationship. Restoring a man's potency in an attempt to save a failing relationship is rarely successful and is more likely to make things worse.

7.5.2 Treatment of ED

ED in diabetes is usually irreversible and most impotent men will require a pharmacological or physical treatment in order to restore potency. Although concomitant antihypertensive medication could be contributing to the ED, anecdotal experience has shown that changing medication is a fruitless activity unless there is a clear temporal relationship between starting the medication and the onset of the ED.

A wide range of effective treatments is available and they are listed in Box 7.1. Almost all men will prefer a PDE5 inhibitor and the other treatments should be used if these are ineffective or contraindicated.

7.5.3 **PDE5 inhibitors**

PDE5 inhibitors act via the NO pathway (Figure 7.2). During tumescence, there is an increase in the intracellular concentrations of NO which acts via cyclic GMP to produce smooth muscle relaxation. Inhibition of PDE5, which breaks down cGMP, enhances erections under conditions of sexual stimulation. Thus, in theory, these agents only enhance the process of erection if the man is sexually aroused.

Currently, three PDE5 inhibitors are available: sildenafil, vardenafil, and tadalafil. All three are effective in restoring erections in 50% to 60% of diabetic men. Tadalafil differs from the other two PDE5 inhibitors as it has a substantially longer half-life (18 versus 4 h) and a single tablet has the potential to normalize erectile function for 2 days.

There is good evidence that PDE5 inhibitors are safe but restoring sexual function is not completely without risk as, like any physical activity, it can precipitate cardiovascular events in those at risk. Although the absolute risk remains very small, the issue of cardiovascular safety must be addressed in all men before treating ED.

PDE5 inhibitors are contraindicated in the presence of any nitrate therapy (including nicorandil) as the combination can use profound hypotension. Nitrate therapy should not be given within 24 h of taking sildenafil or vardenafil and at least 48 h of taking tadalafil.

The adverse effects of PDE5 inhibitors can largely be predicted from their actions as vasodilators and include headache, flushing, dyspepsia, nasal congestion, and dizziness (9; 11). Abnormal vision occurs in about 6% of men taking sildenafil and may be due to the fact it has some activity against PDE6 which is a retinal isoenzyme. Muscle cramps and back pain appear to be a particular side effect of tadalafil.

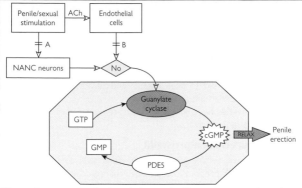

Figure 7.2 Intracellular processes leading to tumescence and pathophysiology of ED in diabetes

Diagramatic representation of pathways leading to and within a corpus cavernosal smooth muscle cell. In diabetes there are defects in NO smooth muscle relaxation due to neuropathy of the NANC fibres (A) and endothelial dysfunction (B).

NO = nitric oxide, NANC = non-adrenergic–non-cholinergic neurons, PDE5 = phosphodiesterase 5, Ach = acetylcholine.

7.5.4 Management of PDE5 non-responsiveness

It is important that men with ED have been appropriately counselled on how to take the medication and have tried at least eight times with a PDE5 inhibitor at the maximum recommended dose before being considered a non-responder.

Hypogonadism should be considered in dealing with men who do not respond as there is some evidence that testosterone replacement in this situation can improve ED as a sole treatment and enhance the response to PDE5 inhibitors. If these measures fail, the patient should be offered a choice of one of the other available treatments.

7.6 Other treatments

7.6.1 Vacuum therapy

Vacuum devices are an inexpensive and effective treatment for ED. Trials in diabetic men have shown that they are effective even in the presence of severe autonomic neuropathy or peripheral vascular disease. Very few serious adverse events have been reported but minor problems are more common, such as bruising and discomfort due to the constriction band or during pumping. Failure to ejaculate can occur in up to one-third of men but anorgasmia is rare. Female partners often report the penis feels cold. Since the advent on oral therapy, vacuum devices have become the forgotten treatment for ED but they remain very effective if the man is willing to use one.

7.6.2 **Intracavernosal injection therapy**

The principle of self-injection therapy is straightforward. Before intercourse the drug (usually alprostadil) is injected into the corpus cavernosum, the penis is massaged and within a few minutes tumescence should occur. It is a highly effective treatment for ED of various aetiologies and can be offered by any physician within a diabetic clinic.

The most important complication of self-injection therapy is priapism which must be treated promptly. Any man using self-injection treatment must be warned to seek urgent medical advice if the erection persists for more than 6 h.

Follow-up studies have shown that long-term usage of self-injection therapy is disappointingly low.

7.6.3 **Transurethral alprostadil**

As an alternative to injection therapy, alprostadil can be delivered *per urethram*. This preparation has been marketed with the acronym 'MUSE®' (medicated urethral system for erection). A placebo-controlled study of 1511 men with ED of mixed aetiology was reported that 65% were able to have intercourse using MUSE®. Penile pain is common and the anecdotal experience of most physicians is that MUSE® has generally been disappointing in diabetic men.

7.6.4 **Other oral agents**

Several agents have been tried as oral treatments for ED. These include yohimbine, phentolamine, apomorphine, and trazodone. The data on all of them is limited and none has stood the test of time.

7.7 **Surgery**

The surgical treatment of ED, in diabetic and non-diabetic men, is usually reserved for those patients in whom more conservative methods have failed or are unacceptable. The most important surgical option remains the insertion of penile prostheses which is effective in appropriately selected patients. A more detailed discussion of the surgical management of ED is best left to more specialist texts (18).

7.8 **Summary**

ED is a common and distressing problem in diabetic men and is easy and rewarding to treat. It is due to failure of NO-mediated smooth muscle relaxation in the erectile tissue secondary to endothelial dysfunction and autonomic neuropathy. PDE5 inhibitors are the first-line treatment and are effective in about 60% of diabetic men.

References

1. Aboseif SR, Lue TF. Hemodynamics of penile erection. *Urol Clin North Am* 1988; **15**(1): 1–7.

2. Alexander WD. The diabetes physician and an assessment and treatment programme for male erectile impotence. *Diabet Med* 1990; **7**: 540–3.

3. Eardley I, Mirone V, Montorsi F et al. An open-label, multicentre, randomized, crossover study comparing sildenafil citrate and tadalafil for treating erectile dysfunction in men naive to phosphodiesterase 5 inhibitor therapy. *BJU Int* 2005; **96**(9): 1323–32.

4. Fonseca V, Seftel A, Denne J, Fredlund P. Impact of diabetes mellitus on the severity of erectile dysfunction and response to treatment: analysis of data from tadalafil clinical trials. *Diabetologia* 2004; **47**(11): 1914–23.

5. Gingell C. The surgical treatment of erectile dysfunction in the diabetic patient. In *Impotence in Diabetes*. Price DE, Alexander WD, Eds. Martin Dunitz, London, 2002; pp. 109–19.

6. Goldstein I, Young JM, Fischer J, Bangerter K, Segerson T, Taylor T. Vardenafil, a new phosphodiesterase type 5 inhibitor, in the treatment of erectile dysfunction in men with diabetes: a multicenter double-blind placebo-controlled fixed-dose study. *Diabetes Care* 2003; **26**(3): 777–83.

7. Jackson G, Betteridge J, Dean J et al. A systematic approach to erectile dysfunction in the cardiovascular patient: a Consensus Statement—update 2002. *Int J Clin Pract* 2002; **56**(9): 663–71.

8. Krane RJ, Goldstein I, Saenz dT, I. Impotence. *N Engl J Med* 1989; **321**(24): 1648–59.

9. Linet OI, Ogring FG. Efficacy and safety of intracavernosal alprostadil in men with erectile dysfunction. *N Engl J Med* 1996; **334**: 873–7.

10. Martin-Morales A, Sanchez-Cruz JJ, Saenz dT, I, Rodriguez-Vela L, Jimenez-Cruz JF, Burgos-Rodriguez R. Prevalence and independent risk factors for erectile dysfunction in Spain: results of the Epidemiologia de la Disfuncion Erectil Masculina Study. *J Urol* 2001; **166**(2): 569–74.

11. McCulloch DK, Campbell IW, Wu FC, Prescott RJ, Clarke BF. The prevalence of diabetic impotence. *Diabetologia* 1980; **18**(4): 279–83.

12. McCulloch DK, Young RJ, Prescott RJ, Campbell IW, Clarke BF. The natural history of impotence in diabetic men. *Diabetologia* 1984; **26**(6): 437–40.

13. McCullough AR, Barada JH, Fawzy A, Guay AT, Hatzichristou D. Achieving treatment optimization with sildenafil citrate (Viagra) in patients with erectile dysfunction. *Urology* 2002; **60**(2 Suppl 2): 28–38.

14. Mulhall JP. Treatment of erectile dysfunction in a hypogonadal male. *Rev Urol* 2004; **6**(Suppl 6): S38–40.

15. Padma-Nathan H, Hellstrom WJ, Kaiser FE et al. Treatment of men with erectile dysfunction with transurethral alprostadil. Medicated Urethral System for Erection (MUSE) Study Group. *N Engl J Med* 1997; **336**(1): 1–7.

16. Price DE, Cooksey G, Jehu D, Bentley S, Hearnshaw JR, Osborn DE. The management of impotence in diabetic men by vacuum tumescence therapy. *Diabet Med* 1991; **8**: 964–7.

17. Price DE, Gingell JC, Gepi-Attee S, Wareham K, Yates P, Boolell M. Sildenafil: study of a novel oral treatment for erectile dysfunction in diabetic men [In Process Citation]. *Diabet Med* 1998; **15**(10): 821–5.

18. Saenz de Tejada I, Goldstein I, Azadzoi K, Krane RJ, Cohen RA. Impaired neurogenic and endothelium-mediated relaxation of penile smooth muscle from diabetic men with impotence. *N Engl J Med* 1989; **320**: 1025–30.

19. Saenz dT, I, Angulo J, Cellek S *et al.* Physiology of erectile function. *J Sex Med* 2004; **1**(3): 254–65.

Chapter 8

Focal and multifocal diabetic neuropathies

Solomon Tesfaye

Key points

- Focal and multifocal neuropathies are relatively uncommon compared to diabetic peripheral neuropathy (DPN) and are unrelated to the presence of other microvascular complications.
- They are characterized by a relatively rapid onset, and complete recovery is usual.
- Proximal motor neuropathy affects patients over the age of 50 and is usually characterized by pain and weakness in the quadriceps. It has a relatively good prognosis with pain resolving within 1 year though residual discomfort may persist for a couple of years.
- The third cranial nerve palsy has a sudden onset but complete recovery is usual.
- Carpal tunnel syndrome is more common in diabetes and treatment involves surgical decompression of the carpel tunnel in the wrist. The long-term outlook to surgery is generally good.

8.1 Introduction

Diabetic peripheral neuropathy (DPN) is the most common manifestation of diabetic polyneuropathy. Less commonly, diabetes can also affect single nerves (mononeuropathy), multiple nerves (mononeuropathy multiplex), or groups of nerve roots. These focal and multifocal neuropathies have a relatively rapid onset, and complete recovery is usual. This contrasts with DPN, where there is usually no improvement in symptoms 5 years after onset. Also, unlike DPN these focal and multifocal neuropathies are unrelated to the presence of other diabetic complications. Asymmetrical (focal) neuropathies are more common in men and predominantly affect older patients. A careful history is mandatory in order to identify any associated symptoms that might point to another cause for the neuropathy. The rapid onset and the focal nature of symptoms suggest a vascular aetiology.

8.2 **Proximal motor neuropathy (amyotrophy)**

Garland was the first to coin the term 'diabetic amyotrophy' to describe this syndrome of progressive asymmetrical proximal leg weakness and atrophy. Other names for this condition include 'proximal motor neuropathy', 'femoral neuropathy', and 'plexopathy'. Typically there is a rapid (within weeks) onset of severe pain that is felt deep in the thigh, but can sometimes be of burning quality and extend below the knee. The pain is unremitting and often causes insomnia and depression. Type 1 and Type 2 patients over the age of 50 are affected. There is an associated marked weight loss that may raise the possibility of an occult malignancy.

On examination there is profound wasting of the quadriceps with marked weakness in these muscle groups, although hip flexors and hip abductors can also be affected (Figure 8.1). Thigh adductors, glutei, and hamstring muscles may also be involved. The profound weakness can lead to difficulty from getting out of a low chair or climbing stairs. The worst affected patients may have complete paralysis. The knee jerk is usually reduced or absent. Sensory loss is unusual, and if present indicates a co-existent distal sensory impairment of DPN.

Figure 8.1 Proximal motor neuropathy (diabetic amyotrophy)

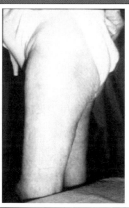

Features

- Older, type 2 male & rapid onset

- Pain, Weakness, paralysis

- Absent reflexes

- Weight loss

- Associated DPN

- Good prognosis

- Tight control of diabetes may help

The diagnosis of proximal motor neuropathy is made by excluding other possible causes of quadriceps wasting such as nerve root and cauda equina lesions, and occult malignancy causing proximal myopathy syndromes such as polymyocytis (Box 8.1). Magnetic resonance imaging (MRI) of the lumbo-sacral spine is mandatory in order to exclude focal nerve root entrapment, malignant infiltration, and other pathologies. Blood tests including erythrocyte sedimentation rate (ESR) and C reactive protein (CRP) level, an X-ray of the lumbar/sacral spine, a chest X-ray and ultrasound of the abdomen may be required. Cerebro-spinal fluid (CSF) protein is usually elevated. Electrophysiological studies may show increased femoral nerve latency and active denervation of affected muscles. Box 8.1 shows the differential diagnosis of proximal motor neuropathy.

The pathogenesis of diabetic proximal motor neuropathy is not known although immune and vascular mechanisms have been suggested. The finding of focal features superimposed on diffuse DPN may suggest vascular damage to the femoral nerve roots, as a cause of this condition.

There is a relatively good prognosis with regard to the pain that usually starts to settle after about 3 months, and usually resolves by 1 year. However, residual discomfort may be present for up to 2 years. Recurrence on the other side is possible but unusual. Motor improvement occurs in the majority although full power may not be regained in some. The knee jerk is restored in 50% of the patients after 2 years.

Management is largely symptomatic and supportive. Patients should be encouraged and reassured that this condition is likely to resolve. The role of tight glycaemic control in the long-term outcome of diabetic proximal motor neuropathy has not been determined by controlled trials although in clinical practice achievement of near normoglycaemia, if necessary with insulin, is recommended. Some patients benefit from physiotherapy that involves extension exercises aimed at strengthening the quadriceps. The management of pain in proximal motor neuropathy is similar to that of painful DPN.

Box 8.1 Differential diagnosis of proximal motor neuropathy

- Spinal cord compression/infiltration
- Nerve root or cauda equina lesion/compression
- Chronic inflammatory demyelinating polyradiculoneuropathy
- Mononeuropathy multiplex
- Focal quadricep myopathy
- Lyme Disease
- Motor neurone disease
- Diabetic amyotrophy
- Occult malignancy

8.3 **Chronic inflammatory demyelinating polyradiculopathy**

Chronic inflammatory demyelinating polyradiculopathy (CIDP) occurs more commonly among patients with diabetes, creating diagnostic and management challenges. Diagnosis of affected diabetic patients is important as CIDP is a treatable condition. There should be a high index of suspicion when an unusually severe, rapid, and progressive polyneuropathy develops in a diabetic patient. Nerve conduction studies show features of demyelination. The presence of three of the following criteria for demyelination is required: partial motor nerve conduction block, reduced motor nerve conduction velocity, prolonged distal motor latencies, and prolonged F-wave latencies. Although electrophysiological parameters are important, these alone cannot be entirely relied upon to differentiate CIDP from diabetic polyneuropathy. Most experts recommend CSF analysis in order to demonstrate the typical findings in this condition: increased protein and a normal or only slightly elevated cell count. However, spinal taps are not mandatory.

The diagnostic value of nerve biopsy is currently a matter of debate. Some authorities assert that nerve biopsy is of no value whilst others consider it essential for the diagnosis and management of up to 60% patients with CIDP. The diagnostic yield of sural nerve biopsies may be limited as the most prominent abnormalities may lie in the proximal segments of the nerve roots or in the motor nerves. Typical appearances include segmental demyelination and remyelination, anion bulbs and inflammatory infiltrates, but these may also be found in diabetic polyneuropathy. A defining feature of CIDP not found in diabetic polyneuropathy is the presence of macrophages in biopsy specimens in association with demyelination.

Treatments for CIDP include intravenous immunoglobulin, plasma exchange, and corticosteroids. Therapy should be started early in order to prevent continuing demyelination and also as it results in rapid and significant reversal of neurological disability.

8.4 **Mononeuropathies**

The commonest cranial mononeuropathy is the third cranial nerve palsy. The patient presents with pain in the orbit, or sometimes with a frontal headache. There is typically ptosis and ophthalmoplegia, although the pupil is usually spared (Figure 8.2). The prognosis is very good and recovery occurs usually within 3 to 6 months. The clinical onset and timescale for recovery, and the focal nature of the lesions on the third cranial nerve in post-mortem studies suggested an

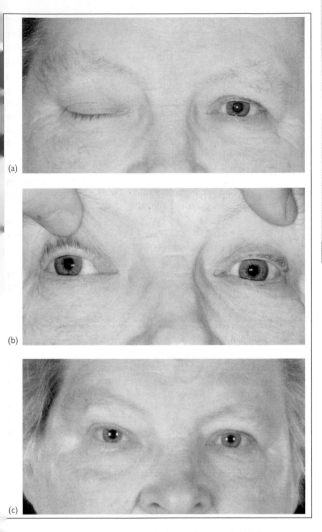

Figure 8.2 A patient with sudden onset third cranial nerve palsy (a) showing ptosis; ophthalmoplegia with mild dilatation of the pupil on manual opening of the eye lid (b), and complete recovery 4 months later (c).

ischaemic cause. It is important to exclude any other cause of third cranial nerve palsy (aneurysm or tumour) by computed tomography (CT) or magnetic resonance (MR) scanning. Fourth, sixth, and seventh cranial nerve palsies have also been described in diabetes but occur less commonly compared to third cranial nerve palsy.

8.5 **Truncal radiculopathy**

Diabetic truncal radiculopathy is characterized by an acute onset pain in a dermatomal distribution over the thorax or the abdomen. The pain is usually asymmetrical, and can cause local bulging of the muscle. There may be patchy sensory loss detected by pinprick and light touch sensory examination. Other causes of nerve root compression should be excluded, and occasionally MRI of the spine may be required. Some patients presenting with abdominal pain as a result of truncal radiculopathy have undergone unnecessary investigations such as barium enema, colonoscopy, and even laparotomy, when the diagnosis could easily have been made by careful clinical history and examination. Recovery is usually the rule within several months, although symptoms can sometimes persist for a few years. Management of the neuropathic pain is the same as the management of painful DPN.

8.6 **Pressure neuropathies**

8.6.1 **Carpal tunnel syndrome**

A number of nerves are vulnerable to pressure damage in diabetes. In the Rochester Diabetic Neuropathy Study, Dyck et al. found electrophysiological evidence of median nerve lesions at the wrist in about 30% of diabetic subjects, although the classic symptoms of carpel tunnel syndrome occurred in less than 10%. Affected patients typically have pain and paraesthesia in the hands that often radiates to the forearm. There is nocturnal exacerbation of symptoms. In advanced cases, examination may reveal a reduced sensation in the median territory in the hands, and wasting of the muscle bulk in the thenar eminence. Median nerve conduction studies show increases median nerve latency confirming the diagnosis. Treatment involves surgical decompression of the carpel tunnel in the wrist. The long-term outlook to surgery is good, although painful symptoms appear to recur more commonly than in the non-diabetic population (18).

8.6.2 **Ulnar nerve and other isolated nerve entrapments**

Ulnar nerve entrapment occurs at the ulnar groove of the elbow. This results in wasting of the dorsal interossei, particularly the first dorsal interossius. Ulnar nerve entrapment is easily confirmed by ulnar electrophysiological studies that localize the lesion to the elbow.

Rarely, patients may present with wrist drop due to radial nerve palsy after prolonged sitting (with pressure over the radial nerve in the back of the arms) while unconscious during hypoglycaemia or asleep after an alcohol binge.

In the lower limbs the common peroneal nerve is the most commonly affected nerve, due to compression at the level of the head of the fibula. This results in foot drop. Unfortunately complete recovery is not usual. Phrenic nerve involvement in association with diabetes has also been described.

References

1. Boulton AJM, Armstrong WD, Scarpello JHB, Ward JD. The natural history of painful diabetic neuropathy—a 4 year study. *Postgrad Med J* 1983; **59**: 556–9.

2. Matikainen E, Juntunen J. Diabetic neuropathy: epidemiological, pathogenetic, and clinical aspects with special emphasis on type 2 diabetes mellitus. *Acta Endocrinol Suppl (Copenh)* 1984; **262**: 89–94.

3. Asbury AK, Aldredge H, Hershberg R, Fisher CM. Oculomotor palsy in diabetes mellitus: a clinicopathological study. *Brain* 1970; **93**: 555–7.

4. Garland H. Diabetic amyotrophy. *Br Med J* 1955; **2**: 1287–90.

5. Coppack SW, Watkins PJ. The natural history of femoral neuropathy. *Q J Med* 1991; **79**: 307–13.

6. Casey EB, Harrison MJG. Diabetic amyotrophy: a follow-up study. *Br Med J* 1972; **1**: 656.

7. Said G, Lacroix C, Lozeron P, Ropert A, Planté V, Adams D. Inflammatory vasculopathy in multifocal diabetic neuropathy. *Brain* 2003; **126**(Pt 2): 376–85.

8. Dyck PJ, Norell JE, Dyck PJ. Microvasculitis and ischemia in diabetic lumbosacral radiculoplexus neuropathy. *Neurology* 1999; **53**(9): 2113–21.

9. Haq RU, Pendlebury WW, Fries TJ, Tandan R. Chronic inflammatory demyelinating polyradiculoneuropathy in diabetic patients. *Muscle Nerve* 2003; **27**: 465–70.

10. Koller H, Kieseier BC, Jander S, Hartung H. Chronic inflammatory demyelinating polyneuropathy. *N Engl J Med* 2005; **352**: 1343–56.

11. Zorilla E, Kozak GP. Ophthalmoplegia in diabetes mellitus. *Ann Intern Med* 1967; **67**: 968–76.

12. Goldstein JE, Cogan DG. Diabetic ophthalmoplegia with special reference to the pupil. *Arch Ophthalmol* 1960; **64**: 592–600.

13. Leslie RDG, Ellis C. Clinical course following diabetic ocular palsy. *Postgrad Med J* 1978; **54**: 791–2.

14. Dreyfuss PM, Hakim S, Adams RD. Diabetic ophthalmoplegia. *Arch Neurol Psychiatry* 1957; **77**: 337–49.

15. Ellenberg M. Diabetic truncal mononeuropathy—a new clinical syndrome. *Diabetes Care* 1978; **1**: 10–13.

16. Boulton AJM, Angus E, Ayyar DR, Weiss R. Diabetic thoracic poly-radiculopathy presenting as abdominal swelling. *Br Med J* 1984; **289**: 798–9.

17. Dyck PJ, Kratz KM, Karnes JL *et al*. The prevalence by staged severity of various types of diabetic neuropathy, retinopathy, and nephropathy in a population-based cohort: the Rochester Diabetic Neuropathy Study. *Neurology* 1993; **43**: 817–24.

18. Clayburgh RH, Beckenbaugh RD, Dobyns JH. Carpel tunnel release in patients with diffuse peripheral neuropathy. *J Hand Surg* 1987; **12A**: 380–3.

19. White JES, Bullock RF, Hudgson P, Home PD, Gibson GJ. Phrenic neuropathy in association with diabetes. *Diabet Med* 1992; **9**: 954–6.

Chapter 9

Management of the diabetic foot

Frank L Bowling and Andrew J M Boulton

Lower extremity pathologies account for more hospital admissions than any other long term medical condition and also results in increased morbidity and mortality

Key points

- Physicians, surgeons, podiatrists, nurses, and orthotists should be integrated into the multidisciplinary team approach.
- Dressings are not recommended in isolation, but should complement debridement and offloading.
- Non-infected neuropathic diabetic foot ulcers will heal without the use of antibiotics.
- A clear understanding of the aetiology and pathogenesis of ulceration is necessary for an accurate diagnosis.
- Ulceration does not occur spontaneously, it is a combination of causative factors.
- Diabetic foot problems result in major medical, social, and economic consequences for patients, their families, and society.
- All patients with diabetes should have a thorough foot examination at least once a year.

9.1 Introduction

he life-time risk of a person with diabetes developing a foot ulcer is stimated to be as high as 25%, and it is believed that every 30 s lower limb is amputated somewhere in the world as a consequence f diabetes (1). The complications associated with diabetic foot disease re set to increase since the contributory factors, such as peripheral europathy and vascular disease, are already present in more than)% of people at the time of diagnosis of Type 2 diabetes.

Up to 50% of amputations and foot ulcers can be prevented by early identification and patient's education necessitating a clear understanding of the aetiology and pathogenesis of ulceration to ensure accurate diagnosis and appropriate treatment. This chapter will focus on diabetic foot complications and its management.

9.2 Aetiopathogenesis of foot ulceration

A clear understanding of the aetiopathogenesis of foot ulceration is essential in order to reduce the incidence and the resulting morbidity and mortality. Foot ulceration is mainly due to neuropathy and/or peripheral vascular disease frequently complicated by a deep-seated infection. Other associated factors are smoking, hyperlipidaemia, sedentary life style, previous ulceration, oedema, foot deformities, callosities, and motor neuropathy. Complications such as retinopathy, renal impairment, microvascular changes, age, gender, and long duration of diabetes are also consistent risk factors for ulceration (Box 9.1). Recurrence is reported in up to 60% of patients with a history of foot ulceration and is common amongst those with more severe complications.

9.3 Clinical examination of the diabetic foot

Careful inspection and examination of both feet is pivotal in the assessment process in order to identify the at-risk foot. A regular foot screen should be carried out annually since amputation is ultimately preventable.

Peripheral neuropathy may be assessed by sensory testing including pinprick, light touch with a 10 g monofilament, vibration with 128 Hz tuning fork and temperature discrimination (Chapter 4). Indicators of autonomic changes can be determined by the presence of warm skin distended dorsal vein, absent sweating, and fissuring of the skin.

Peripheral vascular disease is evident by the presence of cold skin loss of hair, absent foot pulses (dorsalis pedis, posterior tibial), and oedema.

Box 9.1 Risk factors for foot ulceration in diabetes

- Peripheral neuropathy (somatic and autonomic)
- Peripheral vascular disease
- Foot deformity
- Past history of ulceration
- Elderly, living alone
- Previous amputation
- Other microvascular complications (especially if on dialysis for end-stage nephropathy)

If present, any ulcer should be assessed to determine whether it is neuropathic, ischaemic, neuroischaemic, or as a result of pressure necrosis. Previous history of ulceration and infection must be established before any treatment intervention is commenced.

The breadth of classification systems in use reflects the complexity and range of signs/symptoms associated with diabetic foot ulceration. This chapter will use the University of Texas diabetic wound classification system to illustrate the various wound grades (Table 9.1).

9.4 **Prevention**

Regular foot screens and health education should be carried out in the primary care setting. Patients who fall into the low-category fields, that is no identifiable risk factors, should be given general advice on foot hygiene, nail care, and the purchase of suitable footwear. Patients who fall into the high-risk category such as vascular disease, neuropathy, and foot deformities may need a more tailored package to suit their specific requirements. They should be advised on how to wash and inspect their feet on a daily basis. Purchasing of footwear is crucial in the high-risk category and ideally should include wide/deep toe boxes with soft seamless uppers. Barefoot walking should be strongly discouraged due to the risk of traumatic injuries such as foreign objects and thermal injuries. The use of self-treatments should also be discouraged, that is corn plasters, callus removal, and creams containing acid ingredients (keratolytics). Emollients will help to prevent dry skin conditions and fissures and their use should be encouraged on a twice daily basis. Medical attention for any injury or discomfort must be sought directly.

For the patient with a history of recurrent ulceration, podiatric care is of the utmost importance in the prevention of foot ulceration. These patients should be referred directly to the diabetes foot care

Table 9.1 University of Texas diabetic wound assessment classification system

	0	1	2	3
A	Pre- or post-ulcerative lesion (epithelialized)	Superficial, not involving tendon, capsule, or bone	Wound penetrates to tendon or capsule	Penetrates to bone
B	With infection	With infection	With infection	With infection
C	With ischaemia	With ischaemia	With ischaemia	With ischaemia
D	With infection and ischaemia	With infection and ischaemia	With infection and ischaemia	With infection and ischaemia

team. This team should include the diabetologist, podiatrist, nurse, and orthotist: one or two clinicians working in isolation does not constitute a team. Prevention of foot ulceration and subsequent amputation may require the involvement of the orthopaedic or podiatric surgeon to correct deformities such as Charcot foot. The vascular surgeon may be called upon to improve arterial inflow to the lower extremities through bypass grafts and/or peripheral angioplasties.

Optimizing glycaemic control also contributes to the clinical interventions to prevent foot ulceration. The Diabetes Complications and Control Trial (DCCT) reported a 57% reduction in the incidence of neuropathy in patients managed with intensive rather than conventional glycaemic treatment.

9.5 Management of a foot ulcer

9.5.1 Debridement

Diabetic neuropathic foot wounds persist due to disruption of the normal healing process resulting in a sustained inflammatory response. Abnormal values for growth factors have been found within foot wounds alongside abnormal amounts of cytokines and extra-cellular matrix proteins. Matrix metalloproteinase (MMP) levels are reported to be higher than normal in chronic wounds which may be due to overactive synthesis or an imbalance between MMP levels and tissue inhibitors of metalloproteinase (2).

In vitro comparisons of acute and chronic wound fluid have demonstrated that the latter inhibit proliferation and angiogenesis whilst the former actually stimulates proliferation of fibroblasts, keratinocytes, and endothelial cells. It is widely accepted, based on expert opinion, that adequate debridement of wounds is necessary to enhance conditions for healing. The removal of non-viable tissue removes not only the derivatives of the inflammatory response but also any biofilm resident in the wound, thus terminating the chronic wound state to promote healing from an acute state.

The method and degree of debridement selected depends on the aetiopathogenesis, morphology, and clinical presentation of the individual wound but there are essentially four types.

Surgical debridement employs the scalpel blade or other surgical tools to excise non-viable tissue until a firm connection between the epidermis and dermis is displayed. Aggressive debridement with wide exposure can be more effective than minimal incisions in cases of suspected underlying deep infection. Surgical debridement is quick and effective (3).

The principle of autolytic debridement is the facilitation of the body's natural lysis of necrotic tissue by the creation and maintenance of a moist wound bed. This environment is created by moisture retentive dressings but the process as a whole can be slow.

Enzyme-based products have been used to selectively remove non-viable tissue from wounds including collagenase, streptokinase, and streptodornase. Preparations can be in ointment or solution for injection but their efficacy has yet to be established.

Mechanical methods of debridement include the use of wet to dry dressings whereby the wound is hydrated with saline to soften any hard tissue followed by the application of moist dressing. The tissue is left to dry and return to its original hardened state during which time it becomes attached to the gauze. When the gauze is removed the devitalized tissue accompanies it, unfortunately healthy tissue may be at risk and pain is a possibility.

Larvae or more specifically *Lucilia sericata* are extremely effective in removing sloughy necrotic tissue and have re-emerged from the past as a valuable method of wound debridement, having been documented as far back as the 16th century. The excretions/secretions of larvae contain high levels of proteolytic enzymes which function to break down necrotic tissue. This is then consumed by the larvae and as digestion progresses through the gut the bacteria are destroyed. Substances obtained from larvae have been shown to have a high level of antibacterial activity against a range of Gram-positive and Gram-negative pathogens. Samples of larvae secretions have also demonstrated growth inhibition of methicillin-resistant *Staphylococcus aureus* (MRSA) in laboratory settings (4).

Figure 9.1 Removal of larvae from a heel ulcer after they have been *in situ* for 3 days

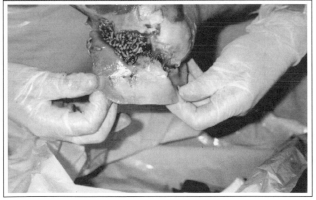

The clinical application of larvae therapy is as an effective method of debridement for sloughy necrotic wounds. Sterile larvae are commercially available from ZooBiotic Ltd. and supplied in half or full pots containing 150 or 300 larvae, respectively. They can be applied directly to the wound or contained in a mesh-like bag. Although the latter is more palatable to patients (and staff), clinical effectiveness is maximized with the former method of application. The wound is then covered with netting and absorbent padding to maintain a moist environment for the larvae to feed.

The application remains in place for a maximum of 3 to 4 days. Additional data is emerging that shows this treatment to be highly effective in reducing MRSA-colonized diabetic foot wounds (5).

9.5.2 **Dressings**

Dressings historically provide a protective covering of wounds shielding them from environmental contaminants. However, modern medicine has attempted to create a multifunctional product that not only protects but also assists the healing process. The range of dressings available is expansive but the evidence base is extremely poor. Diabetic foot ulcers do not lend themselves well to the random clinical trial (RCT) design in view of the diversity in type and presentation whilst the issue is further clouded by the studies available being small in size and often funded by the manufacturers themselves. More recently, data is emerging with improved validity but so far this has examined only acute or non-infected ulcers (Figure 9.1).

Despite lacking a reliable evidence base, the use of dressings makes a frequent contribution to treatment regimes for diabetic foot wounds because at its most basic level a wound will always require some means of protection from the environment. A suitable dressing needs to be impermeable to micro-organisms whilst maintaining adequate oxygenation, capable of absorbing exudate and able to provide thermal insulation. A dressing must be easy to remove without causing damage to the wound itself and demand minimal changes. Beyond these core requirements, there are a plethora of products marketed as offering additions such as debridement, antiseptic/ antimicrobial properties, and facilitation of wound healing. In view of the questionable evidence, base selection will inevitably be based on clinical experience and a solid knowledge of the requirements of wound healing. Dressings are not recommended as monotherapy but should complement debridement and offloading.

Well-known products include honey, silver, and iodine dressings, hydrocolloids, hydrogels and alginates, foams and films, and odour absorbers (Table 9.2).

For an obstinate wound ulcer, sweet wine and a lot of patience should be enough—Hippocrates (460–377 BC)

Table 9.2 Wound management products/preparations

Dressing	Description	Contraindications	Example
Hydrocolloid	Facilitate rehydration and autolytic debridement Dry, sloughy, necrotic wounds Promote granulation	Infected wounds. Twice-weekly change	Aquacel® (Conva Tec) Comfeel® (Coloplast)
Hydrogels	Donates liquid to dry wounds and absorbs exudates Dry, sloughy wounds Autolytic debridement	Hydrogel sheets avoided in infected wounds	Intrasite gel® (S&N) Iodosorb® (S&N)
Silver	Antimicrobial colonization	Sensitivity to silver	Acticoat® (S&N)
Vapour-permeable	Provide a moist healing environment. Mild exude	Heavily exudating wound	Tegaderm® (3M)
Foam dressing	Primary or secondary cover Light and heavy exudates	Remove if strike through occurs	Allevyn® (S&N) Lyofoam® (Medlock)
Odour absorbent	Absorbs odour. Malodorous	Silver (sensitivity)	Actisorb® (J&J)
Larval therapy	Debridement, promote granulation Heavily sloughy necrotic wounds	Increase in pain	(Zoobiotic)
Alginate	Heavy exudates. Blockage	Loose fibres (Advanced Bio Healing)	Kaltostat® (Conva Tec)
Skin substitutes	Obstinate wounds	Infected wound	Dermagraft®
Iodine	Antibacterial. Exudating wounds	Antibacterial. Exudating wounds. Renal/thyroid conditions	Iodosorb® (S&N)
Honey	Antimicrobial. Sloughy necrotic wounds. Autolytic debridement	Medical grade	Mesitran® (Unomedical)

9.5.3 **Skin substitutes**

There are a wide variety of bioengineered tissues commercially available for treatment of acute and chronic wounds. Those with living cells within the matrix are classed as cellular and are sourced from human cells, animal cells, or biomaterials. Dermagraft® is a dermal substitute derived from allogenic, cryopreserved human fibroblasts from neonatal foreskin (6). A polymer mesh acts as a scaffold for the fibroblasts to become confluent, then they begin to secrete growth factors, collagen, fibronectin, glycosaminoglycans, and dermal matrix proteins. The graft begins to act as a living dermal structure and so encourages healing through the in-growth of fibrovascular tissue from the wound bed and re-epithelialization from the wound edges.

Dermagraft® has been used as treatment for diabetic foot ulcers but data regarding effectiveness is limited. It has been compared against saline-moistened gauze and resulted in a greater proportion of patients achieving wound closure in a faster amount of time.

Graftskin (Apligraf®) is derived from keratinocytes and dermal fibroblasts from neonatal foreskin which are then propagated in culture. It is able to produce a number of cytokines and growth factors and angiogenic factors mimicking human skin. When used as treatment for persistent venous ulcers, complete wound closure was achieved at a significantly faster rate than the control. In relation to diabetic foot wounds, a prospective randomized controlled trial compared treatment with Graftskin to treatment with saline-moistened gauze for plantar forefoot neuropathic ulcers. As with Dermagraft®, the results indicated a higher proportion of healed ulcers and faster healing rates in the Graftskin group. However, the major objection to bioengineered tissue products has to be the cost and as yet there is little data to support their widespread use. New studies are required directed specifically at diabetic foot wounds to examine the effectiveness of tissue substitutes against other treatments rather than inert dressings and the cost implications in the long term.

9.5.4 **Negative pressure wound (VAC)™ therapy**

The use of negative pressure to heal complex wounds involves prolonged exposure of the wound to sub-atmospheric pressure via a closed circuit. The commercially available product is the VAC™ or vacuum-assisted closure system. At its most basic level, it consists of a pump attached to an open-celled foam surface dressing which is in turn covered in a transparent adhesive film extending between 3 and 5 cm over the adjacent intact skin in order to provide a seal for the system. The foam is porous so as to ensure even distribution of negative pressure across the wound site. A tube exits the dressing parallel to the wound so as to remove wound discharge and exudate which is collected in an additional canister. Therapeutic pressures can range, but 125 mg Hg may be applied either continuously or intermittently. Dressings are changed every 48 h. Benefits reported include optimization of blood flow through capillary proliferation, increased rate of formulation of granulation tissue, and reduction of tissue oedema (7). The removal of inflammatory by-products contained in exudate supports a moist wound environment. Reduction of bacterial count within the wound and increased epithelialization are also reported. In a clinical context the Vac system has been used with a wide variety of wounds in many different contexts, for example, post-coronary artery bypass grafts on sternal wounds, after raising radial-free forearm flaps, abdominal wounds post-surgery, and skin grafts. The aforementioned are acute wounds but there are also reports of success in chronic wounds such as diabetic foot, pressure ulcers, and venous leg ulcers.

Negative pressure wound therapy as a treatment for diabetic foot wounds has been directly compared with saline gauze, hydrocolloid gel/gauze dressing, moist wound therapy, and advanced moist wound therapy. Results indicated that wounds treated with negative pressure healed in less time and in greater numbers than those receiving the standard treatments (8). A very recent study has also examined additional outcomes including significantly fewer progressions to secondary amputations and no significant difference in complications at 6-month follow-up between groups.

The Vac system appears to offer some advantages over more standard treatments; however, whilst the number of randomized controlled trials appears to be on the increase more RCTs with robust methodology and comparisons with a wider range of treatments would be beneficial.

9.5.5 **Offloading**

Successful treatment of diabetic foot wounds requires attention to the pressures and activity levels to which the wound is exposed (9). Repetitive stress and shear forces play a significant part in ulcer formation; therefore, the redistribution of plantar pressures should be an integral part of any treatment programme. Devices available for offloading are varied and include total contact casts (TCC), removable cast walkers (RCW), and felted foams. The gold standard with a proven track record is the TCC. This is moulded to the individuals' lower limb with limited padding which is in contrast to fracture casts. The aim is to achieve continuous contact with the plantar aspect of the foot and lower leg. The cast remains in place for 1 week but the patient remains able to mobilize. A large number of studies report on its success in comparison to other devices with ~90% of ulcers healed in 6 to 8 weeks. The strength of the TCC lies with the fact that the wound is constantly protected from the forces that created it together with the patient's inability to remove it. Research suggests that non-compliance is high when a removable cast is used with up to 72% of patient activity occurring without the cast. Furthermore, when TCC and RCW are compared the former is more clinically effective than the latter confirming that the success of treatment can be determined by patient compliance.

However, the continuous presence of a cast can have its disadvantages and patients complain of the cast being hot and heavy. Wearing the device can disturb sleep and obviously makes bathing problematic. Other disadvantages include the need for caution in the presence of peripheral neuropathy as symptoms of irritation will likely go unnoticed by the patient and ultimately create new wounds. In addition TCCs are bespoke and therefore require a skilled practitioner and adequate resources to produce, remove, and re-apply as necessary. Despite the above, based on the evidence available the TCC is one of the most reliable methods of offloading and healing diabetic foot wounds.

The RCW attempts to achieve adequate pressure relief whilst counteracting the disadvantages of a non-removable cast. First it is prefabricated thus dispensing with the need for a specialist practitioner for production whilst also being cheaper and easier to replace than its TCC counterpart. The fact that it is removable offers several advantages for both patient and medical professionals. From the patient's perspective it does not offer an obstacle to bathing or sleeping and from the professionals standpoint it allows regular inspection of the wound to assess for infection, monitor healing and debridement as necessary.

Studies have illustrated that the reduction in plantar pressures achieved with a RCW is comparable to that achieved with a TCC but in randomized controlled trials the rate of healing using a TCC far exceeds the RCW (10). An explanation was provided in a study by Armstrong et al. which monitored the activity levels of patients prescribed one of the two treatments and revealed that the RCW devices were worn for the minority of the patients' daily activity (11).

A bridge between the TCC and RCW is the instant total contact cast which involves a simple modification to a RCW to make it non-removable. The result is a cast that is cheaper and easier to provide than a TCC but with equivalent healing times.

Perhaps the simplest form of offloading involves the use of foam padding and felt (12). The felt provides support around the ulcer whilst the foam is used to cover the topical and primary dressing in addition to the felt. Advantages include ease of application and convenience for the patient as standard footwear with a deep toe box will often accommodate the padding. However, healing rates are not as favourable when compared with other offloading devices.

Another pressure relieving option is that of modified footwear such as custom-made sandals, surgical shoes, half shoes, or therapeutic shoes but studies show significantly slower healing times and variable pressure reduction.

Of the offloading methods on offer to the clinician, the TCC provides a level of effectiveness to which all others aspire.

9.5.6 **Antibiotics**

Diabetic patients are ten times more likely than their non-diabetic counterparts to be admitted to hospital for soft tissue and bone infections of the foot. Furthermore, 60% of lower limb amputations in the diabetic population are preceded by an infected foot ulcer (13). Rapid, effective treatment is imperative and requires tailoring to the specific presentation of each individual wound. The bacterial pathogens most commonly associated with diabetic foot ulcers are *S. aureus* and β haemolytic streptococci but these are far from exclusive. Those presenting with recurrent infections previously treated with antibiotics may harbour Gram-negative bacilli within the wound whilst necrotic wounds or those penetrating deeper structures can support both aerobic and anaerobic bacteria. No discussion of infection would be complete without reference to MRSA which has been observed to be increasingly prevalent in diabetic foot wounds (14). Research also illustrates a marked delay in healing when wounds are colonized with MRSA with one study reporting a two fold increase in healing time.

Appropriate antibiotic selection depends on the specific pathogen present and the MRSA climate precludes random selection. Whilst most acute superficial infections, lacking an antibiotic history, can be assumed to be Gram-positive cocci, penetrating infections and chronic wounds may contain multiple pathogens in which case wound cultures will be invaluable in informing treatment selection.

Initial antibiotic choice will depend on the severity of infection and route of administration. Broad spectrum antibiotics are often necessary for major infections or in the interim period awaiting cultures. Treatment against *S. aureus* and streptococci should be included in an initial antibiotic regimen. Culture and sensitivity results may facilitate a change in drug regimen specific to the pathogens isolated. Cephalosporins, for example cephalexin, and the semi-synthetic penicillins such as flucloxacillin may be prescribed for mild to moderate infections. Patients recently treated with antibiotics may require the addition of a fluoroquinolone such as ciprofloxacin to cover the possibility of common Gram-negative bacilli and enterococcus. Severe infections can respond to a second or third generation cephalosporin, for example cefoxitine or ceftazidime, but if there are signs of necrosis antibiotic activity needs to include anaerobes. The later cephalosporins or a fluoroquinolone combined with clindamycin are effective. Severe infections with suspected MRSA will require combination therapy, for example a glycopeptide such as vancomycin or linezolid with a cephalosporin or a fluoroquinolone with metronidazole. The treatments for mild to moderate infections are usually by the oral route whereas delivery of antibiotics for severe infection is parenterally.

9.5.7 **Surgery**

Diabetic foot ulcers are associated with an increased risk of amputation therefore the long-term aim is one of prevention or at least reduce the likelihood of this occurrence. Cases that have failed to respond to the treatments referred to above may require a surgical approach. The patient with diabetes may be considered for surgery for a variety of reasons and at different stages in the ulcer process, but surgical options are explored when the ulcer appears refractory to current treatments and/or is causing significant pain as in the non-neuropathic population (15). For cases where there is no immediate risk to the limb or patient's general health, an elective procedure may be selected as a means of correcting an underlying deformity thus reducing the risk of future ulceration. More radical surgical procedures are required when the viability of a limb is threatened and the risk of a systemic response is high. Once widespread infection and necrosis are present, some level of amputation will be necessary.

Successful surgery is heavily dependent on adequate vascular supply to the affected area; however, revascularization can be performed before osseous reconstruction is carried out.

Achilles tendon lengthening procedures have been advocated to reduce forefoot pressure but this may also be associated with transfer pressure and therefore hold a high propensity for ulcer formation (16).

9.6 **Summary**

The key to reducing morbidity and mortality from diabetic foot disease is the establishment of an active screening service in primary care in order to identify those patients with significant risk factors (17); such individuals then require appropriate education in preventative foot care and more frequent review. Those patients with active ulceration require a detailed assessment addressing the question 'what factors resulted in the development of this lesion?' It then essential to account for all of the causative factors when formulating a treatment plan; it is often more important to ask 'what can I take off this ulcer in order to promote healing'; items such as aggressive debridement and offloading pressure from the ulcer and those most likely to be overlooked. The creation of a foot care team is essential in the overall management of these complex foot wounds.

References

1. Boulton AJM, Vileikyte L, Ragnarson-Tennvall G, Apelqvist J. The global burden of diabetic foot disease. *Lancet* 2005; **366**: 1719–24.

2. Jeffcoate J, Price P, Harding KG. Wound healing and treatments for people with diabetic foot ulcers. *Diabetes Metab Res Rev* 2004; **20**(Suppl 1): 78–89.

3. Boulton AJM, Bowling FL. *Pharmacotherapy of Diabetes, New Developments.* Springer publications, 2007; ISBN-978-0-387-69737-6.

4. Thomas S, Jones M. *Maggots and the Battle Against MRSA.* The Surgical Material Testing Laboratory, Bridgend, 2000.

5. Bowling FL, Salgami EV, Boulton AJM. Larval therapy: a novel treatment in eliminating methicillin-resistant *Staphylococcus aureus* from diabetic foot ulcers. *Diabetes Care* 2007; **30**(2): 370–1.

6. Gentzkow G, Iwasaki SD, Horshon KS. Use of dermagraft, a cultured human dermis, to treat diabetic foot ulcers. *Diabetes Care* 1996; **4**: 350–4.

7. Banwell PE, Teot L. Topical negative pressure (TNP): the evolution of a novel wound therapy. *J Wound Care* 2003; **12**: 22–8.

8. Blume PA, Walters J, Payne W, Ayala J, Lantis J. Comparison of negative pressure wound therapy using vacuum-assisted closure with advanced moist wound therapy in the treatment of diabetic foot ulcers: a multicenter randomized controlled trial. *Diabetes Care* 2008; **31**: 631–6.

9. Armstrong DG, Boulton AJ. Activity monitors: should we begin dosing activity as we dose a drug? *J Am Podiatr Med Assoc* 2001; **91**: 152–3.

10. Armstrong DG, Nguyen HC, Lavery LA, Van Schie CH, Boulton AJM, Harkless LB. Offloading the diabetic foot wound: a randomised clinical trial. *Diabetes Care* 2001; **24**: 1019–22.

11. Armstrong DG, Lavery LA, kimbriel HR, Nixon BP, Boulton AJM. Activity patterns of patients with diabetic foot ulceration: patients with active ulceration may not adhere to a standard pressure off-loading regimen. *Diabetes Care* 2003; **26**: 2595–7.

12. Zimmy S, Meyer MF, Schatz H, Pfohl M. Applied felted foam for plantar pressure relief is an efficient therapy in neuropathic diabetic foot ulcers. *Exp Clin Endocrinol Diabetes* 2002; **110**: 325–8.

13. Pecoraro RE, Rieber GE, Burgess EM. Pathways to diabetic limb amputation. Basis for prevention. *Diabetes Care* 1990; **3**: 513–21.

14. Tentolouris N, Jude EB, Smirnof I, Knowles EA, Boulton AJ. Methicillin-resistant *Staphylococcus aureus*: an increasing problem in a diabetic foot clinic. *Diabet Med* 1999; **6**: 767–71.

15. Hong T, Brodsky J. Surgical treatment of neuropathic ulcerations under the first metatarsal head. *Foot Ankle Clin* 1997; **2**: 57–75.

16. Mueller MJ, Sinacore DR, Hastings MK, Strube MJ, Johnson JE. Effect of Achilles tendon lengthening on neuropathic plantar ulcers. A randomised clinical trial. *J Bone Joint Surg Am* 2003; **85A**: 1436–45.

17. Boulton AJM, Armstrong DG, Albert SF *et al.* The comprehensive Diabetic Foot Exam: report of a task force of the American Diabetes Association. *Diabetes Care* 2008; **31**: 1679–85.

Index